TECHNOLOGY,

BUREAUCRACY,

AND HEALING

IN AMERICA

TECHNOLOGY, BUREAUCRACY, AND HEALING IN AMERICA

A Postmodern Paradigm

By Roger J. Bulger

Introduction by Uwe E. Reinhardt

University of Iowa Press / Iowa City

University of Iowa Press, Iowa City 52242
Printed in the United States of America
First edition, 1988

Library of Congress Cataloging-in-Publication Data

Bulger, Roger J., 1933–
    Technology, bureaucracy, and healing in America: a post-
modern paradigm/by Roger J. Bulger; introduction by Uwe E.
Reinhardt.—1st ed.
        p.   cm.
    Bibliography: p.
    ISBN 0-87745-219-9
    1. Social medicine—United States.   2. Medical care—
United States.   3. Medical technology—United States.
I. Title.
    [DNLM: 1. Delivery of Health Care—Organization & Ad-
ministration—United States.   2. Ethics, Medical—United
States.   3. Health Policy—United States.   4. Technology,
Medical.   W 84 AA1 B93t]
RA418.3.U6B85   1988
362.1′0973—dc19
DNLM/DLC   88-20597
for Library of Congress   CIP

For the memory of my parents, who pushed me toward the best education possible, and my wife, children, and brother, who continually push me to keep learning, even at this relatively late stage. Without these two thrusts, I doubt this book would ever have emerged.

CONTENTS

HEALERS AND BUREAUCRATS
IN THE ALL-AMERICAN
HEALTH CARE FRAY
By Uwe E. Reinhardt

Time was when a troubled medical practitioner would drop by my office once or twice a week on the way home from his practice, there to despair over the latest mischief visited upon mankind by bureaucrats here and abroad.

Often the spotlight was trained upon the evil spirits who guide this nation's Medicare and Medicaid programs. These spirits, it appeared, were bent on destroying "the very best health system in the world." Occasionally the discussion would be more parochial, centering on the latest misdeeds by New Jersey's commissioner of health. Then there was my friend's concern over muckraking researchers who twisted the bureaucrats' minds with papers about unnecessary surgery and diagnostic testing, often in subversive comparisons with medical systems abroad. And always some time would be set aside to deplore the misanthropes at the Food and Drug Administration who touted the economic virtue of generic drugs, in reckless abstraction from the subtle differences in bioavailability that could spell the difference between life and death—differences of which every American physician presumably was fully aware at all times.

In a nutshell, my visitor's laments invariably revolved around one central theme: the serious damage society inflicts upon patients when limits are placed on physicians' clinical freedom to compose medical treatments as they see fit and on their economic freedom to charge whatever honoraria they deem honorable.

So absorbing were our debates on this theme that often I would be home late for supper, as vainly I sought to convince my friend that a nation's resources have many competing uses, and that society at large has a legitimate claim to guide their allocation, including allocations to and within the health care sector.

Came the day when my friend dropped by to decry the latest outrage committed by "socialized medicine."[1] This time the outrage had occurred in the Canadian province of Saskatchewan, which had long covered all of its citizens with a universal government-run health insurance plan. According to my friend, that plan had recently decided not to compensate physicians for elective hysterectomies performed solely to afford patients a preferred life-style. That, argued my friend, was a dangerous intrusion by government into the physician's clinical decisions and demonstrated the ultimate horror to which "socialized medicine" would always descend: the rationing of care.

After about an hour's heated debate, carried on in my office and eventually outside in the street, I had made absolutely no headway with my proposition that, far from interfering directly in clinical decision making, the democratically elected government of Saskatchewan merely had exercised its authority not to pay for care it did not feel obligated to finance with collective funds, and that surely a way could be found by Saskatchewan women to procure this elective procedure as they would procure elective cosmetic surgery.

I was equally unsuccessful in convincing my friend that, in some way or other, health care always has been, was then, and always would be rationed here in the United States and everywhere else on the globe. Some nations, I explained, ration health care overtly by a political process, either through administrative decrees that prohibit the financing of certain procedures or by placing overall limits on the capacity of the health care system. Other countries, including the United States, use the more diffuse method of rationing by price and ability to pay and by the uncertain supply of noblesse oblige among doctors and hospitals willing to treat poor, uninsured patients free of charge. Thus, I argued, the policy in Saskatchewan was just one more instance of rationing certain types of care by price, an approach surely not unknown in our latitudes.

We would probably be arguing that issue still had not my wife driven up at that moment, determined finally to get to the bottom of my stochastic arrivals home. After my plea for her understanding and for her own views on the matter before us, she finally turned to my friend and challenged him with the penultimate question, one every layperson ought to pose to every physician who laments the status quo in contemporary medicine: "In a sentence or two, describe to me your conception of the ideal American health-care system." Whereupon my friend replied, without a moment's hesitation: "In such a system, doctor and patient should be free to select the preferred medical treatment for a given medical condition and someone should pay for that treatment without regulating either doctor or patient." It is literally the only time I have seen my usually graceful wife, a highly educated lady from China's Fujian Province, peel rubber as she sped away in our powerful Cougar, shouting over the engine's roar: "That idea is just too naive to merit my precious time!"

The Youthful Credo of American Medicine

My wife's outburst, albeit a bit candid for that sort of discourse, was right on the mark. Surely there is something outlandish in the idea that society should simply entrust to its doctors and hospitals keys to sundry collective insurance treasuries, there to let these providers fetch for themselves and yet other providers whatever they deem reasonable.

And yet, if I had to distill into a few sentences the vision of a preferred American health system that has been projected to me during some twenty years of health policy debate by physicians in private conversations, by the letters and editorials in medical journals, by the hundreds of resolutions that are debated each year in the American Medical Association's house of delegates, and by spokesmen for organized medicine as they have appeared before the congressionally mandated Physician Payment Review Commission[2] (on which I serve), then that vision would be fairly described by the following credo of American medicine.

A. Health care should be available to all regardless of ability to pay.

B. Only the physician and the patient should determine how to treat the patient's illness.

C. Someone in society should make available, without rancor or second-guessing, the requisite real resources for the treatment chosen by patient and physician.

D. Someone in society should pay the suppliers of these real resources "properly," once again without rancor or questioning fees and charges.

There is something touching about this credo, for it seems so innocent and well intentioned. I say "innocent" because it abstracts completely from the wider social, political, and economic context into which our health care sector must fit—a context that the medical profession may certainly help shape, but one that also inevitably and quite legitimately limits the individual physician's clinical and economic freedom. Having studied the health systems of a number of other nations at closer range, I have come to the conclusion that, while physicians everywhere chafe at the constraints society imposes on them, American physicians are truly unique in the tenacity with which they cling to this youthful credo. It strikes me as one of the major stumbling blocks in our search for a more effective and humane national health policy.

The youthful credo probably was forged during the heady two

to three decades following World War II, when physicians and other health care resources were perceived to be in short supply almost everywhere in this country, and when American society appeared willing to allocate ever-increasing budgets to entice added resources into the health care sector with few questions asked. It was the golden age of medicine in several senses of that term. Assured of a persistent excess demand for their services, American physicians were able to earn a handsome living without having to fight for market share, without having to lean on the advice of marketing specialists, and without having to charge patients and insurers the maximum the traffic would have borne. Consequently, physicians were well appreciated and highly respected by their patients. That respect, in turn, kindled within physicians a high degree of self-esteem.

Perhaps this period of unrestrained growth was long enough to suggest to at least the now older cohorts of the profession that a perfectly abnormal period in the history of medicine was actually a permanent state of nature. Small wonder then that American physicians with a memory of this golden age have found it so difficult to adapt to the newly emerging context, one marked by excess capacity all around, by the need to worry about market share and marketing strategies, and by society's intent to exploit to the payers' advantage the pervasive surplus of health care resources in its many daily bargains with the nation's healers.

Like bright, enterprising teenagers who will not comprehend why even well-to-do parents must, in the end, rein in their energetic offspring—particularly these offsprings' pleas for ever greater weekly allowances—and like teenagers who lapse from time to time into acute depression over such strictures, so have America's physicians struggled in recent years with the growing pains that attend their transition from the abnormal golden age of laissez-faire medicine to a more regular modus operandi under which those who pay for health care also want to have some say.

A good national health policy would guide this transition firmly, but gently, without needless confrontation. A useful first step in that direction would be to explain to practicing physicians precisely what is happening to them and why, just as adolescents are helped in their travails by books that explain to them the bewildering forces that buffet them from within and without.

For teenagers, such books are written by seasoned adults with a keen memory of their own adolescence and thus with the ability to communicate mature ideas in a teenager's idiom. A similarly kind and illuminating literature must come forth for America's bewildered and increasingly paranoid physicians. That literature could possibly be written by sensitive laypersons. More likely, it will be penned by highly educated (as distinct from merely well-trained) physicians with a larger social vision and yet a keen sense of direct patient care. Roger J. Bulger's *Technology, Bureaucracy, and Healing in America*, written by a distinguished American medical practitioner, administrator of several large health care institutions, head of an important national association of medical centers, and frequent participant on study panels or commissions convened to explore aspects of American health policy, is such a book. The book represents a physician's attempt to describe to the laity the agonizing dilemmas practicing physicians encounter at the patient's bedside, but also to understand sympathetically the wider social values and economic forces that create some of these dilemmas.

Dr. Bulger's exploration takes him, in the first three chapters, to a search for an overarching value "by which we can order our affairs, including, of course, our health care efforts." In the end he adds a heightened sense of community to freedom, justice, and hope for the future as that collection of overarching values that should move our society. He concludes that there are, in fact, two sometimes competing sets of values involved in health care delivery: these are embedded in what he refers to as the

"Hippocratic Theme" and the "Bureaucratic Theme." The Hippocratic theme represents a set of moral imperatives that guide the physician at the patient's bedside. One might call it the "micro" or "clinical" ethic of health care. The bureaucratic theme, on the other hand, represents the moral imperatives that guide the overall allocation of society's scarce resources to competing ends, of which health care is but one. We may call it the "macro" or "social" ethic of health care.

These two distinct value systems, argues the author, are coming into increasingly sharper conflict with one another as the modern healer can draw to the patient's bedside an ever-expanding array of sophisticated, expensive technologies. The conflict cries out for a "new, postmodern paradigm" that must accomplish two desiderata. First, it must raise among Americans the value of community—Europeans would call it solidarity—above this nation's much celebrated individualism, which the author finds it hard to distinguish from mere old-fashioned selfishness. At the same time, concludes the author, the new paradigm calls for some amendments to the ancient Hippocratic Oath, to make physicians see beyond the patient's bedside and embrace a broader social perspective.

In the remainder of this essay I shall critically examine the ancient Hippocratic Oath and Dr. Bulger's proposed revisions to it. Next I shall revisit what Dr. Bulger calls the bureaucratic theme from an economist's perspective. Finally, in the concluding sections, I shall comment on Dr. Bulger's vision of a more harmonious postmodern paradigm. While I share his hope for such a paradigm, I am less optimistic than he that such a paradigm can soon, if ever, be achieved. On the contrary, I foresee continued conflict between the "bureaucrats" and the "healers" primarily because we, the people who cheer on both, are so utterly confused about the social role of health care as we switch back and forth from the status of cool and calculating potential patients to the state of being aching and frightened actual patients. No one, of course, adds more to this confusion than economists who, at least while in a state of good health, sincerely seem to believe that individuals who are acutely ill, or their anxious relatives, can be viewed as ordinary "consumers."[3]

The Revised Hippocratic Oath

Let me confess for all to see that I have never been much impressed by the ancient Hippocratic Oath which, according to Dr. Bulger, "remains the bedrock of the commitment made each year by thousands of graduating medical students" in this country.[4] The oath is largely obsolete and it conveys an altogether misleading image of the modern physician.

Among the uninitiated the Hippocratic Oath typically conjures up the image of kindly physicians rendering charity care. In fact "charity care" is not even mentioned in the oath, either explicitly or implicitly. The oath merely affirms the ethical precept of *Primum non nocere* (First, do no harm), the promise not to poison the patient knowingly, the promise to protect the patient's privacy, the promise not to have sexual relations with either patient or relatives[5] (or slaves), the promise not to engage in surgery or to perform abortions,[6] and, finally, the promise to keep the art and privileges of medicine within a carefully circumscribed circle of individuals, chiefly the physician's own male lineage and that of his teacher's.

It would stretch one's imagination to see in the Hippocratic Oath anything about the social ethic that should govern the distribution of physician's services.[7] Nor is there any allusion to the fiscal burden the physician's decisions may impose upon "whatever houses [they] may visit." There certainly is not even the slightest hint about the ethics that should govern a physician's dealings with distant third-party payers, including the government.

Set within the context of antiquity, the Hippocratic Oath may have been a breath of fresh air. Set within the context of modern medicine, however, the oath constitutes a rather limited profession of personal and social ethics. One would wonder just what sustains its popularity among modern physicians, were it not for the romance ancient rituals tend to kindle among the educated in general, and were it not for the felicitous image the oath bestows upon physicians in the eyes of the laity, most of whom probably have not the foggiest notion about what the oath actually does and does not contain. In today's health-speak the oath provides market appeal.

As Dr. Bulger implies, thoughtful persons would respect the medical profession more if it saw fit to abandon its ritualistic allegiance to this largely obsolete oath in favor of the richer, modern version he proposes in chapter 4. In his version Dr. Bulger retains the precepts of *Primum non nocere* and of confidentiality, but he adds a sorely needed stricture on the conflicts of economic interests a physician may ethically shoulder in modern medical practice. Thousands of American physicians already violate that part of Dr. Bulger's modern Hippocratic Oath as they become silent owners of for-profit imaging and rehabilitation centers to which they refer patients, and as they enter into joint ventures with hospitals and lay capitalists.[8]

More important still, Dr. Bulger's revised oath recognizes that, in a modern democracy, physicians help shape the distribution of medical services among members of society in their role both as voting citizens and as voting members in professional associations that seek to purchase preferred health policy outright through so-called political action committees. This particular passage in Dr. Bulger's revised oath is so important that it merits full citation here.

> I shall work with my profession to improve the quality of medical care and to improve the public health. As a citizen, I shall work for equitable health care for all, but I shall not

let other public or professional considerations however important interfere with my primary commitment to provide the best and most appropriate care available to each of my patients.

It can be agreed that every patient—sick bureaucrats and economists included—would wish to have as a physician someone beholden to this ethical precept. Dr. Bulger still lets that precept rest on a slippery slope, however, for he leaves unsaid just who is to determine the limits that must inevitably be placed upon "the best and most appropriate care" made available to the patient and also who is to pay, and how generously, for whatever care is made "available" within those limits. The answers to these two questions constitute the bridge Dr. Bulger seeks to construct between the Hippocratic and the bureaucratic themes. A revised Hippocratic Oath must say more about the structure of that bridge before we can hope for the postmodern paradigm that is to guide American health policy toward greater social harmony. To appreciate how much more needs to be said let us join Dr. Bulger in his sensitive chapter on the bureaucratic theme, but revisit it from the perspective of an economist.

Perspectives on "Resource Allocation in Health Care"

To sympathize with the imperatives that drive the bureaucratic theme it may be useful to start with a glimpse at the statistic at the heart of that theme: the percentage of the Gross National Product (GNP) that is said to be "going to health care" (currently somewhere between 11 and 11.5 percent). What does that statistic actually tell us?

The statistic does not tell us, as seems widely supposed, what real resources (human labor, materials, and so on) are applied in any given year to the treatment of patients. Instead, the statistic merely measures the monetary reward society as a whole bestows upon those who had surrendered these real resources to patient care. In more popular vernacular, we may view it as the slice of that proverbial GNP pie carved out for those who earn their living by participating directly or indirectly in the process of health care, whatever that participation may or may not have done for the well-being of patients.[9]

It follows that the percentage of the GNP going to health care is determined by two factors: (1) the number of health workers— doctors, nurses, other health professionals, clerks and orderlies in health facilities, employees of insurance companies and pharmaceutical firms, civil servants, full-time health economists, and so on—who come to the health care sector to seek fiscal nourishment from the process of health care, and (2) the amount of fiscal nourishment (income) each of these health workers is granted by society.

Now, a fundamental question to be addressed by any coherent vision for an ideal American health care system is this:

> By what process should society decide how many individuals will be permitted to nourish themselves fiscally on the process of health care, and how generous should that fiscal nourishment be for the various categories of "health workers"? Should we apply here the same algorithm free societies tend to use to determine the slice of the GNP going to, say, pizza- or shoemakers? Or should a different algorithm be used, in light of the peculiar nature of health care? If so, precisely what should that algorithm be?

That the algorithm used for pizzas and shoes may not be useful in health care reflects two peculiarities of health care as a commodity which also must be taken as something akin to a state of nature.

First, most modern societies profess the ethical precept that health care should be made available to all who need it, regardless of their ability to pay for it with their own resources (even if that lofty precept is occasionally honored in the breach). This egalitarian principle sets health care apart from ordinary commodities that are permitted to be rationed by price and ability to pay. The precept sets health care apart even from basic commodities such as food, clothes, and shelter for which society is willing to tolerate far greater inequality of access and quality than it seems willing to countenance in health care.

This basic fact of modern health care is one about which every entering medical student in this country should be duly warned, perhaps by having the following inscription chiseled into every medical school's portal:

WARNING!
You are about to enter the terrain of a social good to be distributed on egalitarian precepts. The production and distribution of social goods always involve some government regulation.

Not to warn medical students thus would be irresponsible. On the other hand, having been duly warned, it would be just as irresponsible for physicians to deny a legitimate role for government in health care.

The distinct distributive ethic modern societies impose on health care challenges anyone seeking to propose a vision for the ideal American health system to come to grips with a second fundamental question: precisely to what degree and in what way should Americans be one another's keepers in health care or, to use Dr. Bulger's terminology, what do Americans actually mean by the terms community and nation in connection with health care? It is important to be quite concrete here in the specification of the needed health care that should be available to all members of our nation. For example, is it morally acceptable to deny children of poor families access to preventive services—

say, eye care, dental care, tests for strep throat, and so on—that are readily available to children of well-to-do families? If not, then why has that been the accepted practice in the United States to this very day? And precisely how should access to such services be guaranteed to all?

Next, is it part of our professed (as distinct from practiced) egalitarian precept to make available to all patients newly evolving technology whose efficacy has not yet been convincingly demonstrated? If not, then can one fairly reproach bureaucrats when they deny payment for unproven and possibly harmful new technology? These are troublesome questions, but they ought to be addressed in a revised code of ethics for physicians.

As noted, to effect the egalitarian precept all modern societies apparently seek to impose on health care, government typically must act as insurer of last resort for at least some segments of the population. This circumstance leads to yet another fundamental question: how is the government to compensate those who provide health services to patients in public insurance programs? Many physicians—particularly older ones—dispose of this question with the proposition that, had the government stayed out of the health care sector in the first place, the entire issue of physician reimbursement by government could have been avoided altogether. The assumption here is that private charity would have taken care of the poor and private market forces of the rest. This thesis is usually buttressed with moving stories of decades past when kindly physicians reportedly rendered late-night care in return for chicken and tomatoes, all the while scratching together a modest living from paying patients, through a private tax system called the sliding scale of fees.

Such stories undoubtedly contain a kernel of truth. Hard statistics on the utilization of health services by different income groups before and after the introduction of the Medicare and Medicaid programs, however, show convincingly that, prior to the onset of these programs, the nation's poor had far less access to needed health care than they enjoy now, and less than is suggested by these reminiscences.[10] Furthermore, if American physicians really stood ready to render today's poor all needed care in return for nothing or chicken and tomatoes, then why do they now fuss so much over the low fees paid by Medicaid which, although lower than market, are nevertheless higher than nothing, or chicken, or the fees poor patients could scratch together from their own resources? And why do so many physicians refuse to accept Medicaid patients at all?[11]

Even if the felicitous stories about charity care had once been true in some parts of the country—in rural areas or small towns—in the context of modern-day, expensive, high-tech health care they become dangerous fantasy. There are now some 37 million insured persons in this country, the bulk of whom are poor. Can anyone seriously pretend that so many persons could be adequately served through the unorganized noblesse oblige of doctors and hospitals, particularly in a market that is becoming increasingly price-competitive? Such a fantasy is not only silly, it is downright lethal to poor Americans. It is the opium of a people unwilling to face the realities of modern health care economics.

Let every American physician be reconciled to the fact, then, that somehow the government will always loom large in paying for health services in this country. Thus the question remains how the public sector is to compensate the providers of health care for care rendered to patients in public programs, given that it can never be acceptable for long simply to open the public treasury to let doctors and hospitals take out their "customary and reasonable" scoop without questions asked.

If the government is to pay its healers market rates, it will require much paperwork on the part of both government and providers continuously to establish what the prevailing market is. That is the blight of the present Medicare program as it seeks to determine with much red tape and computer time whether each fee billed by each physician for each service is that physician's usual and customary fee and, if so, whether that fee is reasonable. Uniform fee schedules would be a workable alternative to reduce the paperwork. The question then arises, however, how these schedules ought to be established. Should they be set by the government, or should they be negotiated with associations of providers? Alternatively, should we establish only uniform relative value scales and then have public programs (and private insurers as well) use that scale to elicit from doctors and hospitals truly competitive bids for the monetary conversion factors, coupled with mandatory assignment at the level of the winning bids?

Whatever one's view may be on the matter, a successful bridging of the Hippocratic and the bureaucratic themes requires us to articulate these views clearly, with a detailed plan on the manner by which publicly funded health programs are to be stitched into our private-sector health care quilt. It will not do any longer simply to lament our government as an evil empire presumably not of our making, as remains the medical profession's wont. The empire *is* of our own making, and its mandate from us, the people, to protect our public treasuries will not go away.

Now suppose a supreme power were kind enough to wave a magic wand, thereby removing once and for all the need for government intrusion into health care—perhaps by making us insensitive to the needs of our poor brothers and sisters, so that health care could be rationed simply by price and ability to pay, like ordinary consumer goods. Would the problem of the bureaucrats then go away? Would our healers be free at last?

Clearly the answer is no. The healers would still be left to contend with armies of private-sector bureaucrats bent on constraining the healers' freedom. Even if no one cared about equity in the distribution of health care, the highly uncertain incidence of illness will naturally drive individuals to seek refuge in health insurance pools, not only to smooth out their own outlays for health care over time but also to share with others the risk of financially ruinous illness. But surely a voluntary, private health insurance pool is inherently just as collectivist as a government-run insurance program. Like their public-sector counterparts, the private-sector bureaucrats charged with administering the collective insurance funds obviously must monitor how these funds are spent and control the overall magnitude of that monetary flow. Like their counterparts in government, these private-sector bureaucrats must engage in the much hated cost containment.

At this time, that private bureaucracy reveals itself to America's healers in the form of Health Maintenance Organizations (HMOs), Preferred Provider Organizations (PPOs), Managed Care, and ever-new forms of private-sector intrusions into the practice of medicine. The private-sector bureaucrats who administer these organizations seek to place strict limits upon the best and most appropriate care made available to the physician's patient. More and more these private-sector strictures come to resemble government regulation.

Dr. Bulger's modern Hippocratic Oath does not come to grips with this facet of modern medicine, for his passage on social ethics remains silent on the question of how physicians are to react to the budgetary limits imposed on them by society. Should physicians respect these limits and maximize their patients' benefits within them? Or is it incumbent upon physicians to fight these limits by any means and by any argument, be it truthful or not, on the rationale that all's fair in a war over budgets?

Ever since the onset of the Reagan administration, for example, spokespersons for organized American medicine have deplored the allegedly deep and brutal budget cuts by which that administration is said to have "carved the Medicare program to death slice by slice"[12] with total disregard for the quality of patient care. As early as 1984, New Jersey's daily *Trentonian* was persuaded to that view, for on December 2 of that year the paper scared the aged with a fat, two-inch headline "MDs FEAR SURGERY COULD BE RATIONED." In its issue of February 21, 1986, the American Medical Association's *American Medical News* carried the headline "Medicare Budget Cut $55 Billion in Five Years." A similarly dire message was beamed by a national coalition of hospitals and doctors through advertisements prominently displayed in daily newspapers. In fact, in early February of any year since 1980, just after the president's budget for the coming fiscal year is revealed, most trade journals for doctors and hospitals have featured mournful headlines that decry a new round of painful cuts in the Medicare program.

To the lay public these messages convey the impression that the annual outlay for Medicare has actually been cut year after year since 1980, and that it was therefore much lower in 1986 than it was in 1980. Many practicing physicians, too busy with their patients to dig into the subtleties of published statistics on health care outlays, probably believe that as well, in all sincerity. In absolute dollars, however, total annual outlays by the Medicare program more than doubled during 1980–86, from $35.7 billion in 1980 to $76 billion in 1986! Medicare outlays strictly for physician services almost tripled during that period, from $7.9 billion in 1980 to $19 billion in 1986.[13]

To adjust these data for general price inflation and for the growing number of the aged, figure 1 presents the equivalent data, but restated in dollars of constant general purchasing power and per Medicare enrollee. It is seen that while real GNP per capita rose by about 9 percent during 1980–86 and real health care expenditures per capita for persons under age 65 rose by about 26 percent, real Medicare expenditures per Medicare enrollee rose by over 45 percent and real Medicare payments to physicians per Medicare enrollee rose by over 60 percent.

Figure 1. Increases in GNP and health expenditures in constant 1980 dollars, per capita or Medicare enrollee

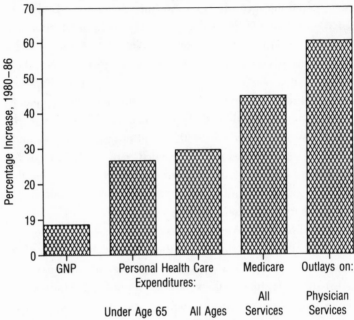

Sources: "National Health Expenditures, 1986–2000," *Health Care Financing Review* 8, no. 4, Summer 1987; tables 10, 15, 16, 17; U.S. Congress, House of Representatives, Committee on Ways and Means, *Background Material and Data on Programs within the Jurisdiction of the Committee on Ways and Means, 1987 Edition*, Washington, D.C.: U.S. Government Printing Office, March 6, 1987; section 4, table 1, p. 139.

In the light of these data, the question surely can be asked on what basis the period 1980–86 can possibly be interpreted as one of brutal budget cuts, of carving up of the Medicare program, and of shrinking resources all around. It would be one thing for physicians to demonstrate convincingly that these sizable increases in real resources were nevertheless still inadequate to support the task at hand. That allegation, of course, would require physicians to explain to the public what had actually been done with the sizable budget increases granted the Medicare program since 1980 and what, specifically, could not be accomplished for want of even higher budget allocations. It is quite another thing, however, simply to step around that demanding demonstration by scaring both the public and busy medical practitioners with the broad allegation that health care budgets were brutally slashed when these budgets actually doubled and tripled in the short span of six years.

Little is gained in the long run if the debate on national health policy proceeds on deliberately distorted images. To be sure, in the short run, that strategy may bring tactical victories over the bureaucrats. But in the long run the strategy is apt to engender cynicism all around and thereby detract from good social policy. The question thus arises, at least in my mind, whether Dr. Bulger's revised code of medical ethics ought not to be amended further to embrace the medical profession's comportment in debates over national health policy. Perhaps that code ought to incorporate, along with the principle of *Primum non nocere* (First, do no harm), also the admirable principle of *Semper veritas!* (Always the truth!). I shall return to this point further on.

The Prospect of a Peaceful "Postmodern Paradigm"

Throughout Dr. Bulger's essay there runs the theme that the postmodern paradigm will reintegrate into a more humane and harmonious whole the three strands of modern health care that he sees at odds with one another: technology, bureaucracy, and healing. Dr. Bulger hopes that this integration will come soon. I am less sanguine on that point.

Indeed, I wonder whether there ever was and ever can be prolonged harmony between a society and its healers, for the latter are never just healers, but partners in commerce as well. No symbol represents this dual role of the healer more admirably than does the ancient caduceus, the familiar herald's staff with one or two snakes coiled about it.

Physicians throughout the ages have looked upon the caduceus as a symbol of wisdom and healing. The traditional caduceus, with two snakes intertwined, is now the official insignia of the Medical Corps of the United States Army. The Aesculapian staff,[14] named for Asklepios (Aesculapius), the Greco-Roman god of medicine, is the official insignia of the American Medical Association.

But the traditional caduceus is also widely known as Mercury's staff, Mercurius being the Roman incarnation of the Greek god Hermes, son of Zeus and Maia, herald of the Olympian gods, and the god of commerce.[15] As Mercury's staff, the caduceus has served throughout the ages as a symbol of commerce as well.

The caduceus thus ably merges the two strands of medicine that trouble not only the soul of the medical profession itself, but also its relationship with the rest of society.[16] That relationship has had some rough edges since time immemorial.

As Chadwick and Mann observe in their *Hippocratic Writings*, "we find plenty of complaints, in both Greek and Roman writers, concerning the greed and cupidity of doctors who are sometimes making colossal fortunes from their gullible patients." In the epistle of St. Luke, chapter 8, verse 42, we read of "a woman having an issue of blood twelve years, which had spent all her living upon physicians." And as early as the 18th century B.C., the Babylonian king Hammurabi felt it necessary to regulate the kingdom's healers by including in the Code of Hammurabi a presumably binding fee schedule.[17] Furthermore, anticipating twentieth-century America only too well, the Code of Hammurabi also prescribed penalties for what was then perceived as medical malpractice. The code, for example, provided that "if a doctor has treated a man with a metal knife for a severe wound, and has caused the man to die, or has opened a man's tumor with a metal knife and destroyed a man's eye, his hands shall be cut off."[18] American physicians, beset by a growing malpractice crisis—one that seems bent upon destroying the relationship of trust and goodwill between patient and healer—may wonder how Babylonian society coped with its own malpractice code.

The ambivalence and tension inherent in the relationship between society and its healers are unlikely ever to vanish, for the herald's staff carried by the healers switches forever back and forth between its Aesculapian and Mercurian versions, in a manner that both confuses and rankles the laity. At the patient's bedside, physicians typically carry the Aesculapian staff in their role as healers in the Hippocratian mold. In that role, and as individuals, physicians usually earn the respect and the affection of their patients—even of patients who would not extend these sentiments to the medical profession as a whole.

The medical profession seeks to project the Aesculapian version of the caduceus also in its dealings with third-party payers or regulatory commissions. It does so by converting absolutely every discussion on budgets and fees (or any debate on professional licensure)[19] into the issue of the quality of patient care. Alas, as the path-breaking work of John H. Wennberg[20] has demonstrated, there is as yet great uncertainty among physicians over what constitutes high-quality health care. So far, the profession has not been able to explain why the use of health services by seemingly similar populations and the per capita cost of health care vary as enormously as they now do across regions in this country. These inexplicable variations in practice patterns, and a newly emerging literature on the apparently pervasive inappropriate application of medical and surgical procedures to patients,[21] cast doubt on the profession's claim that there exists a tight correlation between health care expenditures and the quality of health care.

Sooner or later the Aesculapian imagery projected by physicians in these forums tends to wear thin, to reveal the caduceus' Mercurian spirit. Inevitably, as already noted earlier, that denouement breeds cynicism all around. As a member of the previously cited Physician Payment Review Commission, I have always been saddened to see a proud and otherwise admirable profession expose itself thus to cynicism and ridicule. How much better it would be for all concerned if physicians were willing to discuss in these forums their quite legitimate economic aspirations, citing threats to the quality of care only when the causal link between budget and quality can be convincingly specified. I would view such candor a matter of professional honor and as the *sine qua non* of the postmodern paradigm Dr. Bulger espouses. In that spirit, I propose that he add to his revised Hippocratic Oath the following codicil:

> I promise to state facts truthfully, as best I know them, in public debates over health care budgets and over my professional fees. Furthermore, I promise never to hide behind the shield of "quality of care" in defense purely of my own or my profession's economic interests, unless there demonstrably exists a clear causal link between those economic interests and the quality of patients' care.

That codicil would not in any way prevent American physicians from defending their incomes in discussions with patients or third-party payers, as physicians in other countries openly do, without thereby losing society's respect.[22] Nor would it prevent physicians from alerting bureaucrats to sincerely perceived threats to the quality of health care available to patients. It would merely put physicians on guard against confusing their own economic interests with their patients' welfare, a confusion that might lose them society's respect.

Uwe E. Reinhardt

Strategies and Tactics for the All-American Health Care Fray

No one can fairly deny that behind the fantastic technological innovations in modern medicine described by Dr. Bulger there lies the inventor's and the healer's urge to help suffering fellow human beings. But no one would foolishly deny that behind these also lies the awesome force of commerce—the economic aspirations of countless business enterprises who see in health care one of the richest and most rapidly expanding American frontiers and who see in the economic aspirations of healer-entrepreneurs[23] the stuff for a powerful economic alliance.[24]

Locked in step, this army of lay and professional entrepreneurs now marches on toward the jagged perimeter defended by the motley crew of private- and public-sector bureaucrats charged with defending our sundry insurance treasuries. Behind these valiant guards camp we, the people, cheering on either side of the fray, depending upon our health at the time.

In the status of healthy consumers who purchase insurance policies, of employee-benefit managers of business firms who purchase insurance or health care on their employees' behalf, of politicians who must appropriate funds for public health care programs, and of taxpayers whose funds are so being appropriated we cheer on the bureaucrats and berate them every time they surrender territory to the armada of healer-entrepreneurs. But in our role as frightened and aching patients or their relatives, we are easily persuaded by the armada's heralds that the armada and its high-tech armamentarium carry relief and that only mindless and heartless bureaucrats stand between us and that relief. Thus, we cheer on the armada and curse the bureaucrats for every victory they seek. It is an unseemly and confusing battle, one that will last a long time and may go on forever, for the battle of commerce is rarely tranquil, and it is often rough. The business of healing, amounting to over half a trillion dollars now and growing rapidly year after year, will be no exception.

In seeking to defend our collective treasuries from unwanted inroads by the healers, the bureaucrats assigned to that thankless task can pursue one of two broad strategies, and countless mixtures in between. The choice among them is, of course, not only the bureaucrats'. It is largely determined by the strategies and tactics adopted by the advancing army.

At one extreme, the bureaucrats may content themselves simply with placing overall budget limits upon the healers, entrusting to the latters' managerial acumen the task of procuring with these funds an appropriate mix of real health care inputs, and leaving to the healers' clinical judgment the allocation of the services produced with these inputs. In its purest form, that is the approach taken by the British National Health Service and by its American cousin, the Health Maintenance Organization. It is also increasingly being adopted in the hitherto more loosely structured Canadian, French, and West German national health insurance systems.[25]

At the other extreme, if the bureaucrats cannot somehow impose upon the healers an overall budget constraint *ex ante*, then they will sooner or later be driven to control their outlays on an ongoing basis, by monitoring each and every transaction for which they pay—that is, by second guessing both the providers' clinical and pricing decisions. That is the approach increasingly being taken in the United States, where managed care, the control over the physician's clinical judgments, goes hand in hand with competitive or regulatory pressures on the prices for individual health services.

American physicians should not miss the irony inherent in the strategy to which they have acquiesced, wittingly or unwittingly. After having led the good fight against the economic shackles inherent in universal national health insurance—that is, against the overall budget constraints and fee schedules such systems tend to impose upon the healers—they now find themselves surrounded by lay emissaries from a myriad of public and private payers, each seeking to influence both the physician's prices and his or her medical treatments. As Dr. Bulger notes in his chapter 5, European and Canadian physicians would be appalled at the numerous intrusions into clinical decisions now routinely made by these external monitors in the United States. They probably would rise up in arms over that loss in clinical autonomy.

Yet, remarkably, American physicians seem to put up with the intrusion—albeit unhappily—in their tenacious fight to preserve the individual physician's right to price his or her services as they see fit. I have drawn attention to this irony so often during meetings of the Physician Payment Review Commission that its members have kindly come to refer to it as Reinhardt's law. A concise rendition of that law might read like this: in modern health care systems, the preservation of the healers' economic freedom appears to come at the price of their clinical freedom.

The micromanagement of medical treatments by external managers grows daily in this country. It now involves such tactics as preadmission authorization for proposed admissions of patients to the hospital, concurrent external review of patients in the hospital, and *ex post* review of patients' charts, and it goes so far as to trigger, from Medicare, letters to both doctor and patient, announcing that this or that particular medical procedure applied by the physician in a particular case was judged by Medicare, *ex post*, as medically unnecessary and that, therefore, the physician owes the patient a refund of any fee already paid. Once again, it can be doubted that Canadian and European physicians would tolerate this intrusion directly into the doctor-patient relationship.

So continues the all-American health care fray, now and in

the foreseeable future. One must assume that, bright as the nation's physicians are, they knew full well what they were doing when they let our health policy slip into this grand strategy— when they gambled away their clinical freedom to preserve their economic freedom. Presumably, at the time, the price paid was considered worth the prize gained, and perhaps that loss of complete clinical freedom will in the end work for good for the patient and healer. If not, then let Dr. Bulger and kindred spirits show us a better way, lest, by default, that way be paved largely by our valiant bureaucrats.

Notes

1. Actually, the term "socialized medicine" is confusing. One should distinguish "socialized financing of health care" from "socialized production of health care." In England, Sweden, the socialist countries, and in the U.S. military there are both socialized financing and production of health care. Under the national health insurance system of, say, Canada, only the financing of health care is fully socialized. Health care is produced by a mixture of publicly owned and purely private facilities, just as it is in the United States.

2. The commission was established by Congress in 1985 to advise it on policies on the payment of physicians under the federal Medicare program. Represented on the commission are six physicians and a variety of health policy analysts.

3. In any given year, between 75 and 80 percent of all health care expenditures are accounted for by only about 10 percent of the population who, presumably, are quite sick. To model these and their relatives as rational consumers takes considerable imagination.

4. The oath is presented in full at the beginning of chapter 4.

5. Are physicians actually excised from their profession for that infraction?

6. These strictures are actually at variance with the practices of the Hippocratic school whose writings, the *Hippocratic Corpus*, deal ex-

plicitly with methods of surgery and abortion. In this connection, see Albert S. Lyons, M.D., and R. Joseph Petrucelli II, M.D., *Medicine* (New York: Harry N. Abrams, 1978), pp. 214–15.

7. In *Precepts*, a later treatise included in the *Hippocratic Corpus*, doctors are admonished not to succumb to avarice, to consider the patient's means when fixing fees, and, on occasion, to render charity care. But one must wonder how many modern medical students have read *Precepts*, let alone swear allegiance to its dicta. In any event, the Hippocratic Oath itself does not contain any such strictures. In this connection, see J. Chadwick and W. N. Mann, *Hippocratic Writings* (New York: Pelican Books, 1978), especially the introduction by G. E. R. Lloyd.

8. For an exploration of these trends, see Arnold S. Relman and Uwe E. Reinhardt, "Debating For-Profit Medicine and the Ethics of Physicians," *Health Affairs* (Summer 1986): 5–31.

9. In this connection, see Uwe Reinhardt, "Resource Allocation in Health Care: The Allocation of Lifestyles to Providers," *The Milbank Quarterly* 65, no. 2 (1987): 153–76.

10. See, for example, David Rogers, *Statement before the Senate Subcommittee on Health and Scientific Research*, U.S. Congress, Senate Committee on Labor and Human Resources, September 24, 1980.

11. I would be the last to argue that physicians are obliged to render the poor care free of charge. Doctors and hospitals should always be adequately compensated for such care. I am merely contesting the proposition that doctors and hospitals would have taken care of the problem if only the government had stayed out of health care altogether.

12. See, for example, the American Medical Association's *American Medical News*, January 9, 1988, p. 9.

13. See "National Health Expenditures, 1986–2000," in *Health Care Financing Review* 8, no. 4 (Summer 1987): tables 15 and 17.

14. This version has one snake coiling about a staff.

15. Among the Olympian gods, Hermes appears to have held a rather rich portfolio of protectorates. Along with being the god of commerce, he was the god of science and invention, of eloquence, of cunning, and of trickery and thievery as well.

16. In this connection, see Arnold S. Relman and Uwe E. Reinhardt, *op. cit.*

17. The relative value scale underlying this fee schedule reflected the relative worth of the patient being treated. For example, if a doctor had treated a freeman with a metal knife for a severe wound and cured him, the fee was ten shekels of silver (a very high sum by those days' standards). If the patient was only a plebeian, the prescribed fee was five shekels of silver. If the patient was a slave, the owner paid the physician two shekels of silver. See Lyons and Petrucelli, *op. cit.*, p. 67.

18. Lyons and Petrucelli, *op. cit.*, p. 67.

19. Mandatory licensure that excludes nonphysicians—e.g., pediatric or geriatric nurse practitioners—from diagnosing and treating patients is almost always defended by physicians with appeal to the quality of care. Economists have never been much impressed with that argument and see in that defense instead mere protection of economic turf. In this connection, see Milton Friedman, "Occupational Licensure," in his *Capitalism and Freedom* (Chicago: University of Chicago Press, 1981), and Paul J. Feldstein, "The Political Economy of Health Care," in his *Health Care Economics* (New York: John Wiley and Sons, 1979).

20. See, for example, John Wennberg and Alan Gittelsohn, "Small Area Variations in Health Care Delivery," *Scientific American* 246, no. 4 (April 1982): 120–34, and Philip Caper, "The Physician's Role," in Frank B. McArdle, ed., *The Changing Health Care Market* (Washington, D.C.: Employee Benefit Research Institute, 1987), pp. 33–36.

21. The journal *Health Affairs*, Spring 1988, contains a series of papers on this issue. See, in particular, Kathleen N. Lohr, Karl D. Yordy, and Samuel O. Thier, "Current Issues in Quality of Care" (pp. 5–18), David M. Eddy and John Billings, "The Quality of Medical Evidence" (pp. 19–32), and Philip Caper, "Defining Quality in Medical Care" (pp. 49–61).

22. In light of the incomes earned by other professionals—especially the lawyers who torment physicians so in malpractice litigation—it would not at all be difficult to defend the current average

incomes earned by American physicians with appeal either to value added or equity.

23. Although a certain percentage of American physicians could not fairly be described as entrepreneurs, the great bulk of them are and, indeed, take great pride in their "free enterprise" spirit.

24. One need only examine, for example, the medium through which the manufacturers of diagnostic equipment now alert physicians to the profit potential in office-based laboratory equipment. One recent advertisement unabashedly advertised such equipment with the symbol of a goose laying a golden egg and with the words "A golden opportunity to maximize your returns from diagnostic testing." Another refers to "Quick-Profits" through "Quick-Chem." Yet another apprises the physician that a new piece of equipment is "a money maker for the physician," and so on.

25. Although, as noted, these systems socialize merely the financing of health care and not necessarily its production, they increasingly place overall budgetary limits upon the funds that may be disbursed to providers. Since 1985, for example, the West German sickness funds have transferred to physician associations fixed overall budgets which are then distributed to individual physicians on a fee-for-service basis.

PREFACE

I owe a great deal to the Tanner Lecture Series for starting me on the road to the effort which has led to this book. I must, at the outset, express my deep appreciation to Dr. Benjy Brooks for recommending my name to the Tanner Selection Committee at Clare Hall, Cambridge University. The Tanner Lectures are an endowed series of lectures to be presented annually at each of four American and British universities on the general subject of ethics and society. At Clare Hall, the Tanner Committee gave Professor Patrick Echlin the task of organizing the lectureship according to a new format, to which I agreed with enthusiasm. The plan was to give me two years to prepare a series of four lectures on health care and human values. These lectures were presented over two days but had been submitted for preliminary reading by selected American and British experts who served as commentators at an all-day symposium, which took place on the third day. The public was invited to participate fully in the proceedings of the third day, and it was a great privilege to have had Sir George Godber, the first director of the National Health Service, in attendance and adding his insights on several occasions. The American participants were Professor Robert Veatch, Kennedy Institute of Ethics, Georgetown University, Washington, D.C. and Alexander M. Capron, Topping Professor of Law, Medicine and Public Policy, University of Southern California—Los Angeles. Both of them made deep and searching criticisms of my lectures and have, I am certain, influenced my subsequent handling of that same material and the additional substance of this book, which was not a part of the

Tanner material. I thank them deeply and sincerely for their contribution to this book through their efforts in Cambridge, England in the spring of 1987.

As always seems to be the case, however, it seems as though one can learn the most from strangers, especially strangers who come from a different culture but whose speech is intelligible. British colleagues, through the prism of their differing perspectives, invariably can stimulate Americans to look a little more sharply at their own enterprise and their own understandings of their own enterprise. This was done ably by the Right Honorable Lord Byron Hunter of Newington; Bryan Jennett, M.D., dean and faculty professor of medicine, University of Glasgow; Ian Kennedy, Kings College, London; Mr. Robert Maxwell, King Edward's Hospital Fund for London; and Mr. Paul Sieghart, Gray's Inn, London. I must, however, single out Bryan Jennett, a famous surgeon who is most provocative on the question of technology assessment and whose work should be read by every American concerned with health care delivery. The experience of spending two weeks at Clare Hall and discussing the major health care issues with so many people knowledgeable about the National Health Service was of incomparable help, because nothing else can emphasize the magnitude of the pride of the British in the fairness of their system, the equality of access it provides to all citizens, the independence and autonomy on professional matters still maintained by their doctors, and their frustrations over the shortfalls in services that deficiencies in funding necessitate.

A previous extended visit to the United Kingdom with the attendant opportunities to interview officials of the National Health Service and practitioners of medicine allowed me to get a good general feeling for the reactions of the British experts to the ideas that were emerging in my mind. Since these lectures were to focus on American health care and seemed likely to get significant international exposure, I wanted to be certain that my lectures fairly represented the American health care scene; thus, I circulated the four manuscripts to over twenty American experts in medicine, health, or health policy and benefited from their commentaries, incorporating many of their suggestions in the final lectures. Therefore, some of their ideas and thinking may also be in parts of the current book and, though I cannot blame them for the book's deficiencies, I thank them heartily for making many helpful suggestions which have led to substantive improvements. Their names follow: William W. Bulger, Ruth Ellen Bulger, Wilbur J. Cohen, Barbara Culliton, Bradford Gray, Lawrence Green, John Hogness, George R. Kerr, Darwin R. Labarthe, Walter J. McNerney, Sam A. Nixon, Edmund Pellegrino, Uwe E. Reinhardt, Stanley Reiser, Julius Richmond, L. Rodney Rogers, Steven A. Schroeder, Anne R. Somers, Larry Tancredi, Sam Thier, and Karl D. Yordy. A sharply condensed version of the four lectures is being published in the latest annual volume of *The Tanner Lectures on Human Values* by the University of Utah Press.

Since my return from England, I have worked on the development of the manuscript which has resulted in this book, and, although in concept and in some details my thinking has changed and evolved, there is no doubt that the majority of the impetus for this volume is owed to the Tanner Lectureship.

I owe many thanks to Leslie Reedy, who patiently typed and prepared the many drafts of the manuscript, to Louise Milliner, who carefully guided, from the author's end, the treatment of the many necessary details that arise at the interface between author and publisher, and to Mary Jane Dennis and Mary Bulmahn for their backup support. Finally, we all owe a debt of gratitude to my friend Henry Fung, whose cover illustration summarizes the main point of this book better than the proverbial one thousand words.

Preface

I owe special thanks to the Regents and to my superiors in the University of Texas System for allowing me the opportunity to develop this manuscript while serving as the chief executive officer of the University of Texas Health Science Center at Houston.

I am especially indebted to my friend Uwe Reinhardt. I asked him to write an introduction, because all books need an introduction; but I asked him to apply his economist's perspective to the issues I raise as a citizen and a physician. I asked him to be as critical of my views as he could be, because I felt the reader would benefit by getting the economist's counterpoint right away. He has succeeded fully in rising to that challenge—so much so that I wondered whether to place his essay at the end, as a kind of summary, instead of at the beginning.

Finally, I decided to keep it an introduction, but I recommend that serious readers go through the essay a second time, after they have finished the rest of the book. I suggest this not because it allows Professor Reinhardt both the first and the last words, or because he says so much with which I agree, but because it puts in the parentheses of economic reality my perhaps romantic, even quixotic hope for a new postmodern paradigm.

In the end, it is for the reader and, of course, the public to decide which of us is right.

TECHNOLOGY,

BUREAUCRACY,

AND HEALING

IN AMERICA

1 SOCIETAL AND PERSONAL BIASES

This is a time of incredible flux, of volatility and paradox in America's health care industry. Just when we have achieved almost unimaginable technological advances, with science moving forward on both the basic and applied fronts, we begin to experience deep and searching doubts about the value of technology in general. Just when we thought that we had conquered the infectious diseases and the genetic diseases were about to fall, along comes the AIDS epidemic to give a further boost to molecular research and to remind us that our level of ignorance far exceeds our level of knowledge. Just when our society was beginning to take pride in its progressively improving record in providing access to care for all our population, we take steps which are associated with a tendency to reverse that progress. Just when organized medicine thought it had avoided the specter of health care managed by the federal government through a national health insurance program, forces are unleashed which seem to be promoting a health care enterprise dominated by large institutions or corporations which, from the providers' point of view, may be as nefariously bureaucratic as the federal government threatened to be. Just when patients most need doctors they can trust to help guide them sensitively through the technological mine field of options confronting them, the medical liability crisis has developed to the point where a doctor-patient encounter is seen by both parties as adversarial rather than covenantal. Just when it seems that our technologies have so engulfed us that the human and personal elements of compassion are no longer cost beneficial in the health care transaction, the neurochemical revolution occurs to show us how emotions and environment can cause us to alter our own brain chemistry so that the doctor can potentially help us cure ourselves through the establishment of a relationship, through something other than introducing a pill, a procedure, or an operative intervention. Just when it seemed that psychiatry and the rest of medicine might never meet, the valid interface between behavioral and molecular medicine is convincingly explored by investigators examining the placebo effect, the relaxation response, and a host of other mind-body interactions.

To put the matter differently, just when it seemed that the fragile confederation of technology, bureaucracy, and the person of the healer had come apart, with each going its own way, according to the late twentieth-century American reductionist approach, as exemplified in the seemingly sterile and meaningless anomie of our overweening affluence, there are signs of a change toward a new postmodern paradigm based on a new ordering of our values which could reintegrate the three strands (technology, bureaucracy, and healing) in a new, more humane, and more effective approach to health care.

America thought it could perhaps make death only an option through the seemingly never-ending stream of new miracle cures that have tumbled out of our research laboratories over the last thirty-five years, but we now understand that technology brings its own suffering, that we shall soon be confronting an epidemic in chronic, long-term care for an unprecedentedly large army of elderly people. The age of unending material and technical progress has passed and in its place we have enshrined the bottom line, the gestalt which promotes the view that the right economic incentives shall set us free or at least control our costs and promote efficiency.

Now, though, we hear increasingly the stirrings, out of sadness, of desire for a new sense of community, a new sense of societal direction that can give meaning to our lives and our problems, that can infuse our efforts at efficiency and economy with a sense of purpose, that can, in effect, explore and develop a new set of transcendent values by which we can order our affairs, including, of course, our health care efforts. As a reasonably well-educated citizen, I have felt, over the past decade, a coming together of different intellectual disciplines, a movement toward a kind of new sense of intellectual unity. Physicists seem to talk almost like theologians; cosmologies rise and fall but emerge almost uniformly now on a scale that seems to equal that of Thomas Aquinas or Karl Barth or Teilhard de Chardin (the priest Teilhard de Chardin proclaimed that he was never closer to God than when he was engaged in active scientific research). At a less rarified level, more and more people are questioning the singular concentration on the reductionist approach which has led us to know and learn more and more about less and less, which has led us to the knowledge and then the technology that can literally destroy us through nuclear immolation. More of us, only recently aware of the bicameral nature of our brains, are appreciative of the fact that the left hemisphere isn't enough; science, organization, and logic can make order and progress, but mystery, beauty, and love can make life meaningful and vital. The right hemisphere and indeed the deep subconscious, where presumably the myths, instincts, primitive drives, and wisdom lie encoded in their DNA from thousands and millions of years ago, all serve to inform and enlighten our existence, if only we can tap them. In short, more and more of us, while not eschewing the benefits of reductionism, appreciate the need for more integration, for a greater sense of the whole, and in our modern democracy a heightened and more functional sense of community. We want our scientists and we want our economists, but neither is enough; together they do not fulfill us, even if they can partially explain us and our behavior. We sense that there is more, and we are looking for it with a new openness and a new energy.

Out of this cauldron, we all hope, a new postmodern paradigm will emerge that can move us as a people—and surely then our health care will follow. It may be that just because health care is so personal, so intensely meaningful for each of us, that working out our values through our approach to health care may, in fact, serve to facilitate our societal effort at a new conceptualization of society itself and its future and direction.

As a society, we have been concealing from ourselves that we are, in fact, rationing our health services. As an Israeli expert and colleague puts it, "In the U.S.A., you ration by price, while in Israel and England, we ration by queue! You pay not to wait, while we wait not to pay!" So others recognize the stark reality of rationing in their countries and in ours; we as a people cannot much longer delude ourselves on this point.

We must now make decisions about who will get how much of what in health care. How much technology and for whom? How much human caring and human and social support for the poor, the children, the elderly, for all of us? And the price is mind-boggling, thus making mandatory our need for making decisions that we'd rather defer or avoid indefinitely. The tendency to treat health care as a business and its problems and dilemmas as business problems and dilemmas amenable ultimately to the strategies of industrial and management techniques is a serious misjudgment. In health care, we are dealing also with some of the most important of our society's values and touching our deepest human concerns as individuals.

My humanist friends frequently identify Hayden White's book *Metahistory* as among the most important of modern times, because in it he analyzes the work of four brilliant nineteenth-century historians, all of whom considered themselves objective observers, and White argues convincingly that each wrote from a distinct point of view which altered his perceptions. In fact, it can be argued that no one, even a natural or physical scientist, is free from observer bias, heavily influenced by the current belief paradigm. Thus, it seems appropriate for me to offer the reader a little of my own background and experiences, especially those which may bear upon or reflect the prism through which I see our health care world.

As a boy of six, I got an acute bacterial pharyngitis and pneumonia and knew that everyone expected me to die. I remember Dr. Cirillo preparing to perform a tracheotomy, which seemed to help me for quite a while, allowing the new wonder drug sulfanilamide a chance to kill all the evil, invading organisms. I remember a kind man, Dr. Shapiro, sitting by the bed and watching me for an hour at a time, apparently wishing me through my illness. I remember my parents being in the room when the tracheotomy clogged up, causing my father to rush out and grab a passing doctor who, in turn, saved me from asphyxiation. I remember too an extraordinary episode, wherein my father was placed supine on a table a foot or so higher than mine in the transfusion room so that blood could flow directly from his veins into mine. When I recovered, there is no wonder then that I felt I owed my life to the combination of a new chemotherapeutic agent, a surgical intervention, two doctors, a bunch of nurses, and my family. In my view, they all operated together to effect a cure; no one of them alone did the job.

I went to medical school intent on becoming a practitioner of medicine, chose internal medicine as the vehicle, and spent more than a decade deeply involved in taking care of patients, public and private, acutely and chronically ill. I trained in internal medicine at the University of Washington in Seattle, just at the time when chronic hemodialysis was being introduced and perfected there. We all regarded the new technique as virtually miraculous, for there was no doubt that these people were brought back from the brink of certain death; yet there was a message also in the shocking decision by one of my patients not to accept the offer to go on chronic hemodialysis. The woman who turned down the privilege of becoming a chronic dialysis patient stunned us all because we had all been hoping she would be accepted. She was extremely mature and relatively young; but after consultation with her family she chose not to live the rest of her life chained to that machine. Her intelligence and courage affected all of us who knew her, but we learned that not everyone wants to live regardless of the cost.

On the other hand, there were many stark lessons in rationing at that time in Seattle when an anonymous lay board decided which patients would receive the limited hemodialysis resource on a chronic basis. The most difficult case for many of us was that of the beautiful sixteen-year-old woman who was stricken with acute and permanent renal failure, which turned out to be due to systemic lupus erythematosis and which, therefore, made her a less optimal candidate than we had thought and hoped. She had to be sent home to die because there was no room for her, a difficult pill to swallow for all those who had worked so hard to save her life; but the pill was far less bitter than if we had had to make the rationing decision ourselves rather than being her advocate as we had been to the deciding board.

Working at a leading university hospital for a decade, and with advanced training in both nephrology and infectious diseases, I was privileged to be able to work with and successfully use some of the most spectacularly successful new diagnostic and therapeutic tools. However, I learned some other lessons through experience. My father had become a chiropractor in his early forties and when I went to medical school he taught me a technique he used to relax tense muscles by pressing steadily and firmly on the insertions of the involved muscle. Once when I was called to see a severely hypertensive nun, a college president who had come in with an excruciating headache, I was able to put my father's technique to good use. In those days we had much less in the way of drug therapy to fight hypertension and we feared the severe headache because it frequently meant the onset of the dread complication of hypertensive encephalopathy.

This intelligent and high-powered person was well aware of the significance of a severe headache for her. After looking in her eye grounds with my ophthalmoscope, I knew she did not have encephalopathy; I was then free to use my father's technique, which in fact completely relieved her headache (along with the knowledge that she didn't have encephalopathy) within fifteen minutes. The laying on of hands is not always only symbolic. She asked me how I did it. I told her it was a miracle, but to go her way and tell no one! She knew not to take me seriously and was a good student as I tried to teach her how to relax her own muscles.

Later, as my professional emphasis switched to an administrative concentration, I learned how seductive technology can be in support of institutional financial well-being. Those of us who have been close to health care over the past thirty years have been able to observe how hard it has become to use technology sensibly and sensitively, especially when it comes to trying to stop a technique once it has been implemented.

Along the way, I spent four years working on health policy matters at the Institute of Medicine of the National Academy of Sciences and received a midlife liberal education from lawyers, economists, public officials, and behavioral scientists, as well as other health professionals and medical scientists. Thus, I came to see more clearly that health care is intimately intertwined with and embedded in the basic values of the society and culture it serves and represents.

From an educational standpoint, the most profoundly useful and productive year of my life came when I delayed medical school to spend a year at Cambridge University in England. Although it is extremely difficult to be certain that one knows deeply anything about another culture, it is certain that continuing exposure yields ever more useful comparisons with one's own culture, one's own values, practices, and strategies. This is especially true if the other culture shares basic values but is sufficiently different and remote to be nonthreatening. All these characteristics are true of cross-cultural studies with England. For this reason, I believe that continuing comparisons between the United Kingdom and the United States will bear fruit in the area of health care and public health policy. Thus, recent studies like those by Americans Henry Aaron and William Schwartz (1984) and England's Bryan Jennett (1986) must be continued, because their value is not to inform the other culture about what it ought to deliver but to add some perspective on what one's own culture ought to be doing.

I have worked in five major medical centers and lived for prolonged periods in my adult life in five different sections of the United States after having spent one illuminating year in England. In England I came to understand why I was an American and preferred to be an American, and I have subsequently learned that, although there is a clear-cut commonality in values in all the places I have lived, there are also very distinct and important differences which create sectional flavors and regional approaches to major issues which simply must be understood and may too easily be ignored. As we strive in America for a national sense of community, we shall have to understand and respect the differences among the regions and the many people whose lives are intensely affected by regional forces and influences. East and west, north and south, and the heartland of America's middle all represent differing gestalts and those differences, in general, should be respected and celebrated; we should not, as a nation, seek to make national policies out of values which reflect only the majority of people in particular sections unless the issue is clearly one of national priority.

It is out of this mind-set, these biases, prejudices, and experiences, that this book has been conceived, developed, and written. These few comments will provide the reader with some sense of where my biases are and foreshadow several of the points detailed later.

2

THE
VOLUNTARY
SOCIETY AND
ITS VALUES

The dog starved at his master's gate
Predicts the ruin of the State!
—William Blake

It is my purpose to reflect upon the current status of
health care and health policy in the United States, exploring
some essential human values considerations with an eye toward
the future and the possibility of attaining the highest quality humanistic health care. In this attempt to ascertain where we
Americans have been in health care delivery, where we are, and
where we might be going, there will be ample opportunity for me
to make comparisons with the situation in the United Kingdom.
However, I shall not yield unduly to those temptations, trusting
that the several scholars who have taken on aspects of trans-
cultural health care will accept the challenge of comparative ex-
aminations of the British system. Many Americans have what I
call the Alexis de Tocqueville syndrome, which is founded in
deep envy of that wonderful Frenchman who came to America in
the mid nineteenth century and described it peerlessly. The patient, suffering from the Tocqueville syndrome, is characterized
by an extraordinary certainty that he or she fully understands
another culture or another nation after having been there for a
few weeks or months or even years. The most severely afflicted
believe they know how to solve all the major problems in the
other country and are annoyingly outspoken in their efforts to
enunciate those solutions for all to hear. During the year I spent
as a university student in England in 1955 I received a perma-

nent immunization to the Tocqueville syndrome. Thus, I trust the reader will understand why I shall limit myself to occasional observations about differences in health care between England and the United States and shall leave the value judgments and things I don't know about to others.

If there is to be an examination through the human values prism of health care in our democratic society, there must first be an exploration of the values which drive the nation in general.

Max Weber, the nineteenth-century German social scientist, taught us that modern societies are evolving bureaucratically in their attempts to rationalize the technological fruits of science. The institutions that emerge in the ever more complicated evolution of modern societies are driven by core ideas which provide institutional cohesion and direction. The bureaucratic pressures, according to Weber, will always be toward greater centralization. We shall return later to this idea that society is driven to organize in such a way as to deliver most effectively the fruits of science; let it suffice for the moment to declare the importance of this idea to our considerations.

Kingman Brewster, in his Tanner Lecture at Cambridge University in 1980, spoke of "The Voluntary Society" (a term which refers to modern democratic states, especially, in this view, England and the United States and defined the purpose of the state to "be to permit life to be as voluntary as possible for its citizen." Freedom for the individual, I think we would all agree, is an essential fundamental for both our nations and the essential cornerstone for the United States.

The one hundredth anniversary of the Statue of Liberty was celebrated in 1986, and that occasion stimulated a Theodore White article in the *New York Times Magazine* in which White wrote about "The American Idea" as follows:

The idea was there at the very beginning, well before Thomas Jefferson put it into words . . .

"We hold these truths to be self-evident, that all men are
created equal, that they are endowed by their creator with
certain inalienable rights, that among these are life, liberty
and the pursuit of happiness."

But, over a century-and-a-half (since 1620 when the Pil-
grims landed), the new world changed these Europeans,
above all the Englishmen who had come to North America.
Neither King nor Court nor church could stretch over the
ocean to the wild continent. To survive, the first emigrants
had to learn to govern themselves. But the freedom of the wil-
derness whetted their appetites for more freedoms.

Mr. White went on to point out that the American nation was
born of an idea, not a place in which families had existed for
time out of mind; he indicated that that idea of life, liberty, and
the pursuit of happiness, as it did in the beginning, continues to
mean different things to different Americans, although all would
agree to its centrality to their society.

This tradition of individual direction and freedom makes the
Anglo-American experience, according to Brewster, distinctive
in all the world. But for a life to be truly voluntary, as Ralph
Dahrendorf (1979) has shown, "ligatures" are as important as
choice. "Ligatures" refer to those ties to family, craft, profession, location, or class which provide a voluntarily held connection to an idea or entity, which in turn gives meaning or a sense
of belonging to individuals in a free society. England and America have both emphasized ligatures and choice in their pursuits
of a voluntary society, but the Americans have emphasized
choice through mobility with rather less concern for ligatures
than the English, where ligatures have been primary often at the
expense of mobility.

Brewster then asks, "How does a society which has relied
upon mobility to keep life voluntary react when the promise of
mobility begins to fade?" Surely this question goes to the heart

of the angst and cultural anomie which have characterized American society in recent decades; meaninglessness begets self-destructive behavior, whether it be expressed in alcohol, drugs, or violence to self or others. He leaves it "to others more intimately experienced to address themselves to the equally interesting query of how a society which has relied upon ligatures to keep life voluntary should react when the ligaments of family, community, craft, and calling begin to lose their ability to bind."

The freedom of the individual remains the dominant value in our society, taking precedence over several other values, including, for example (at the present time in the United States), universal access to good health care.

It can be argued (not compellingly from my point of view) that individual freedom is not the dominant value expressed through the British and American versions of the voluntary society; it is certainly correct that it is not the only important fundamental value of our societies; and it may be that many of our most thoughtful citizens wish it weren't so and argue cogently and convincingly for a more appropriate balancing of responsibility and a sense of community with our commitment to individual freedom. The fact remains, however, that progress toward equal access to health care is not being achieved in the United States and that most people in the United States apparently do not now regard health care as a right. The individual's freedom has a purpose, though; it is linked to a commitment to some serious work. In this regard, Thomas Merton, the famous Trappist monk, wrote about learning to live as follows (1979):

> Life consists in learning to live on one's own, spontaneous, freewheeling: to do this one must recognize what is one's own—be familiar and at home with oneself. This means basically learning who one is, and learning what one has to offer to the contemporary world, and then learning how to make that offering valid . . .

The world is, therefore, more real in proportion as the people in it are able to be more fully and more humanly alive: that is to say, better able to make a lucid and conscious use of their freedom. Basically, this freedom must consist first of all in the capacity to choose their own lives, to find themselves on the deepest possible level. A superficial freedom to wander aimlessly here or there, to taste this or that, to make a choice of distractions (in Pascal's sense) is simply a sham. It claims to be a freedom of "choice" when it has evaded the basic task of discovering who it is that chooses. It is not free because it is unwilling to face the risk of self-discovery . . .

This description will be recognized at once as unconventional and, in fact, monastic. To put it in even more outrageous terms, the function of the university is to help men and women save their souls and, in so doing, to save their society: from what? From the hell of meaninglessness, of obsession, of complex artifice, of systematic lying, of criminal evasions and neglects, of self-destructive futilities.

It may be noted at this point that Americans created their government out of a dislike of central authority; the Constitution is full of distrust for power in the central government. Equally important to this distrust, however, is the drive to conquer misery.

As American historian Oscar Handlin pointed out (1973), peasants from Europe were often wretched aliens in the ghettos in which they landed after a tough passage, but none of them expected their children to die where they were born or to share in the misery of their parents. Even now, from all over the world, emigrants to the United States are repeating that drama; my daughter's college roommate came to America a dozen years ago from Hong Kong with her parents and grandmother. Among her family members, only my daughter's roommate and her brother speak English, but the older generation came to give the younger one a chance at freedom and opportunity through education. In 1987, on a visit to the Holy Land, in the town of Nazareth, I bought orange juice from an Arab street vendor who squeezed the oranges individually upon receiving one's order. He told of his son, whose picture he showed us, who had gone to America for college and dental school and was now practicing dentistry in North Carolina. At a recent graduation from the United States Air Force Academy, the choice for the number one graduate was one of the Vietnamese "boat people" who had come to America at age fourteen. So the hope is still being fulfilled. It requires the fierce independence of a competent individual to break the cycle of inherited, perpetual misery, which effort, many astute observers believe, is the most central feature of American life. If one accepts this as a fundamental characteristic of our nation's development, it is easy to understand modern America's reliance on mobility, on the fresh start and the second chance, and easier still to understand the translation of those emotive forces into many of the health policy decisions that have been made in recent years.

Various forces have tended to make dependent citizens instead of competent citizens of our people. The development of or tendency toward the welfare or entitlement state is one such force, and the professionalization and specialization of society, such that individuals need help to solve everyday problems, is another. The growing narcissism in our materialistic society is a third force that tends to describe a citizenry less inclined to work for a common good, to work for an ideal shared by the larger society, and more inclined to seek the short-term satisfaction of individual desires.

Brewster shared the anxiety of many thoughtful observers when he worried about a purposeless society. Without the promise of purpose, there is little in the American prospect likely to give us heart. Put another way, in a negative cast, he asked, "Most particularly, can America avoid becoming an increasingly resentful society as it faces the realities of pervasive government, ever-larger and increasingly impersonal private business and financial organizations, barriers to mobility imposed by specialization, and both physical and social limits to growth?"

Although it might seem strange for Kingman Brewster, Oscar Handlin, and Ralph Dahrendorf to be linked with Thomas Merton, they all express the fundamental dimensions of the concepts of individual freedom which move our voluntary societies: freedom to choose our own way as individual citizens; hope arising from the opportunity always to begin again, to find a new path, to recover; responsibility to preserve these values for those who follow; and dedication to give something back to the society. In my view, any health care enterprise of the future that aspires to be true to our American values must be true to these basic roots of our culture. That is to say, humanistic health care for the twenty-first century in the American version of a voluntary society must begin with the idea of allowing the individual to fulfill his or her potential as a person, of providing freedom of choice wherever possible, and of keeping alive the hope of a new beginning, repair, or reconstruction. Currently, the concept of fairness, or equal access, seems of lesser importance than the first three but may gain in stature if its impact upon the first three can be demonstrated to the public or if a new dimension, a postmodern paradigm for society and health care, can gain popular acceptance.

This idea of the possibility of a new set of governing ideas (or additions to our existing set such that our governing ideas are collectively altered so as to influence and alter our sense of societal direction and our actions as a society) is introduced at this point because of the pessimism, as expressed by Brewster, that the ligatures which hold our society together as "voluntary" can long maintain their effectiveness in that regard. Things seem to be coming unglued; our old rules don't seem to rule anymore and individual expression seems unrestrained and sometimes ungovernable. There is a growing unease with our current ways, an enlarging sense of directionlessness, a loss of connectedness, a need for community and for a rationale or concept that can help us feel comfortable once again as citizens of our nation and our world. Certainly, we can say we lack somewhat the sense of community and social purpose that was characteristic of the people John Winthrop and Thomas Jefferson helped lead; such is an important value element we lack. We shall return to this issue later, when a possible postmodern paradigm is discussed.

Having thus identified the principal societal values which should be considered fundamental in the development of health policies, let us now turn to the great ideas shaping the modern health enterprise in Western democracies. I have chosen to group these ideas within one of two major themes to be considered: (1) the theme of the healer, which can be referred to as the Hippocratic theme, and (2) the theme of the organizing and financing of the delivery of health services, which will be referred to as the bureaucratic theme. It is my belief that the values inherent in the Hippocratic theme are coming increasingly into conflict with the values inherent in the bureaucratic theme. I shall discuss each of these themes separately in an effort to better understand and articulate the thematic values essential to each. It will then be easier to understand the nature and anticipate the seriousness of conflicts arising out of value clashes emanating from these two roots.

It might be well to digress briefly from the main flow of the argument to clarify the selection of the term *Hippocratic theme*, because the name of Hippocrates can suggest a variety of characteristics. The choice of Hippocrates, instead of, say, Florence Nightingale, after whom to name this theme is based upon the conviction that that name should suggest Western, scientific medicine, a patient-centered commitment on the part of the health professional to which he or she has been bound by an oath, and a tradition of compassion and kindness which, at its origin, sought to treat a person rather than an illness. The sexism, paternalism, and particular restrictions of the Hippocratic Oath are seen by me as phenomena of the times and should not be accepted as indestructibly eternal baggage on the Hippocratic train as it moves through the twentieth to the twenty-first century. Using the Hippocratic tradition tends to lead us to focus upon doctors and to appear as though we are ignoring dentists, nurses, and other health professionals. It is not intended to be thus; on the contrary, the team of health care professionals, captained usually by the doctor but increasingly by other health professionals, is becoming more and more of a widespread reality. The nurse, for example, is the heart and soul of care giving in the modern hospital even though the doctor calls the diagnostic and therapeutic shots. Thus, if the reader will grant me a little poetic license in my choice of Hippocratic theme and try to understand my points in a broader context of all the healing professions, it will undoubtedly save time and prevent confusion.

Central to the bureaucratic theme over the next decade will be an ongoing debate over how to allocate scarce resources. Increasingly, some commentators refer to "rationing" of health care and claim that it is already going on. This is such an important issue that it will be discussed in Chapter 6. The book *Tragic Choices*, co-authored by Guido Calabresi and Philip Bobbitt (1978), develops what to me is the most fruitful approach to the conceptualization of the issues involved.

It will be suggested that as our society resolves these thematic value conflicts in evolving its system of health care, there must be care taken not to undermine those underlying societal values with which we began this discussion. I sometimes make these abstract considerations more tangible in my own mind by envisioning a quadrilateral discussion involving Thomas Jefferson (representing the basic values of the voluntary society), Hippocrates (representing the modern scientific healer), and Max Weber and Guido Calabresi (representing together the bureaucratic imperative).

If American policy makers could hire Jefferson, Hippocrates, Weber, and Calabresi to serve as consultants to meet, review, and discuss our health care policies and actions once each year for the next decade, we might improve our decisions. If some of my guesses about the future are correct, I would strongly recommend adding Robert Bellah (who, with his colleagues, has written an important new book on the sense of community, individualism, and commitment in modern America) to the group. This recommendation will be explained and clarified in subsequent chapters. If we could add to the group as two senior staff one health care expert each from England and the United States, then we might anticipate an even more fruitful consultation. England and America can best help each other not by seeking to convert the opposite number to a different way but by openly comparing what each does and what is or is not working. Thus I shall end up advocating periodic serious comparative reviews, from the human values perspective of health policies in the two countries, as a constructive, ongoing activity.

3

THE HEALTH CARE SCENE IN MODERN AMERICA WITH SOME BRITISH COMPARISONS

Since so much of our American society has its roots, directly or indirectly, in Great Britain, it is natural for the two countries to compare their performances in the health fields. Such comparisons can be entirely constructive if they are rendered with candor and directness but with a clear understanding that what is right or feels right for one country is not necessarily right for the other. Alternatively, what would be judged immoral, inappropriate, or downright stupid in one country should not necessarily be judged so if carried on in the other. It is all too tempting for experts to view another country in the light of their own nation's values, standards, and contexts; in such settings, outspoken, albeit honest, criticisms may do more harm than good, whereas a thoughtful factual comparison may yield a better understanding of the values underlying each nation's health behaviors, which in turn can leave the citizens of each nation to come to their own conclusions and to act accordingly.

A good example of the differences can be illustrated by overlaying a map of the United Kingdom on the United States. England fits neatly into a land mass equal perhaps to Iowa, Kansas, and Missouri; all the nations of western Europe would fit easily into the continental United States. Surely no one is surprised that the twenty or so countries of Europe have twenty different health care systems with widely varying performances in health outcomes or in health care practices; but when we find variations among, for example, surgical practice standards from region to region in America, we find it very upsetting, because we expect almost machine-tooled uniformity.

Although we share a common language and so many other cultural traits and practices, it remains nevertheless correct that there are important, generalizable differences. The British are more orderly, more community oriented, more accepting of long lines for service, less likely to move from job to job and city to city. Americans tend to be more technology oriented, more likely to take action in a difficult situation even if there is no evidence the action will do any good, and more prone to play the angles to "beat the system" to the benefit of the resourceful individual. I have a British friend who characterizes Americans as people who regard death as an option, whereas most Americans express amazement at the tolerance and patience of British patients as they wait for months and even years for certain elective procedures.

In order to set the stage more fully, let me with some trepidation go deeper with these generalizations about health care in the two countries. I shall not dwell upon the dramatically rapid installation in the United Kingdom of the National Health Service (NHS), which essentially from its inception has provided comprehensive health care for 90 percent of the population; the small minority gets its care in the private sector. The NHS has been politically popular from the beginning and remains so with the great majority of Britons, despite growing complaints about excessive waiting times for some services and a generalized, occasionally critical shortfall in finances. This form of organization for the delivery of health services is fair, providing the entire population with equal access to available care; it is economical, spending about half the percentage of the gross national product (GNP) on health as we do in the United States; it is (paradoxically) less intrusive than we have become in the United States into the professional prerogatives of doctors and health professionals in determining the content of health care practice; it is more closely attuned to local citizen desires in that after a sum of money is allocated to a district the local board determines how it shall be expended; and it is more integrative of all the necessary health services since it considers dental services, home care, nursing homes, drugs and protheses, and rehabilitation.

The observation is frequently made that the British devote 6 percent of their GNP to health care while we dedicate 11 percent, and yet we can find very little difference in the measurable health statistics characterizing the health status of the two populations. In 1984, 41 percent (or about 4.5 percent of our GNP) of our total health expenditures came from the public treasury, whereas almost 90 percent (or in excess of 5 percent of the GNP) of the United Kingdom's health expenditures came from public sources. No other country among the Western democracies spent more than 8.9 percent of its GNP on health in 1984, so there is no denying we spend more on health in this country than anywhere else in the world.

The nature of these higher costs will be discussed later, but there is no doubt they have something to do with our penchant for high technology and our desire to fix things that can be fixed and to delay death, perhaps forever. One extremely knowledgeable British physician, Bryan Jennett, marshals a good deal of evidence to show that in those instances where an expensive technology is used more pervasively in the United States than in the United Kingdom, it has not been shown to be a truly effective technology in terms of enhancing length and quality of life. Supporting his view is a recent American study of mortality among patients admitted to either an academic physician or community physician with the same illnesses and the same degrees of severity of disease. The cost of the care rendered by the academic physicians was considerably higher than that rendered by the community physicians, but the hospital mortality was lower. At discharge, 70 percent of the faculty's patients were alive, while 50 percent of the community physicians' patients were alive. Three months later, only 35 percent of the faculty's patients were surviving, while 30 percent of the community phy-

sicians' patients had survived; after eight months, the lines con-
verged such that 20 percent of each group survived for one year
after discharge. This study took place in the same hospital and
included forty-eight matched pairs of patients admitted one to
each service. Among the possible interpretations of the data is
that the technology-intensive care provided by the full-time faculty, with a cost in excess of that provided by community-based
physicians, had short-lived benefits. Such data fit in with Dr.
Jennett's general view of American medicine: we use too much
technology too often and in situations wherein its effectiveness
has not been proven or is so short-lived as not to be worth the
extra cost.

The fact that we spent, in 1984, over \$1,600 per person on
health care compared to the \$600 spent in England has turned
the spotlight on American technology use and procedural interventions. A spate of well-documented studies has made clear
that there are dramatic, unexplained regional variations in certain surgical procedures and in expensive interventions like
coronary angiography (which, in 1982, was done half as often in
the western part of the United States as in the South); furthermore, patterns of practice between neighboring communities
can vary significantly. All of this is contributing to a rising tide
of doubt and uncertainty in the public mind regarding the cost-
benefit ratio of what we're doing in America.

British medical students and physicians, after visiting with
their American colleagues, seem frequently to feel uncomfortable with our relative lack of reliance upon the history and the
physical exam, the time-honored basics of clinical practice.
They are even more uncomfortable with our over-reliance upon
expensive and far too numerous laboratory tests and procedures.
They observe that their American counterparts work under many
more bureaucratic constraints on a day-to-day, hour-by-hour
basis. There is no doubt that most of the British people I have
met seem to prefer the British situation to the American one.

It is equally true, however, that most Americans who have experienced both systems would opt for ours. American reactions to our problems are in general that we must improve, that we have lost ground on cost control and access and equity issues, but that we still have the best medical care available in the world. American patients would not tolerate the long waits for specialty services, nor would most of them be happy to have their care dictated by a gatekeeper primary physician. If an American patient wants to go to an oral surgeon or ophthalmologist, he or she won't often accept an intermediary, especially if the answer is negative. American doctors who visit the United Kingdom sometimes note that the discontinuity between the gatekeeper who cares for patients outside the hospital and the specialists who care for them in the hospital can produce some disadvantageous results. In America, doctors tend to care for their patients in and out of the hospital, increasingly operate in multispecialty groups, and tend less than their British counterparts to use effectively all the society's resources available for the patient's benefit. British primary care doctors tend still to practice alone and therefore are less likely to know as much about what a specialist knows and when the specialist would do one or the' other maneuver. Hence, our doctors are more comfortable doing more things of a specialized nature, and it would be a mistake to think we in America could be satisfied adopting the British approach in its entirety. Thoughtful American critics of American practice habits believe we could cut 25 percent of our laboratory testing without losing anything on the quality side. There are proportionately many more specialists than generalists practicing in America than in the United Kingdom. Americans seldom leave their own city to get specialty care and it is a rarity for an American to leave the country for care.

Aaron and Schwartz (1984), in analyzing British data, conclude that the British underutilize some treatments and technologies and must, in effect, ration their use in situations we couldn't accept in America. I introduce these matters not for the purpose of taking sides on controversial issues or to lead the reader to any conclusion other than that comparisons of these two friendly countries can yield important and penetrating questions that should gain our attention.

To raise difficult questions does not mean we are doing poorly. In fact, the seemingly endless cost comparisons between America's health care and that of other Western democracies frequently obscure the many great successes of the American public health establishment in health promotion and disease prevention. A recent report from the surgeon general on the status of the health goals for the nation in 1990 elaborated the extraordinary detail of our health promotional strategies and the remarkable success in achieving many of our specific goals years ahead of the targeted date. A similar report of the National Health Service shows that the United States compares well in many areas, or that in some areas, quite surprisingly, the United Kingdom is lagging too far behind, such as in the incidence of smoking.

We have discussed the extent and depth of the British commitment to health care for all and have implied that there is a difference in the American view. In the Great Society of the mid 1960s, health care was proclaimed a "right," but in fact it has never attained that status. In a recent study conducted by Arthur Andersen Co. of attitudes of panels of health administrators, health professionals, and patients, 83 percent of all respondents either strongly or slightly disagreed with the proposition that "the entire U.S. population is entitled to the same level of health care." Later, we shall explore these issues in greater depth, but it is an essential difference in the approaches to health care in the two nations. It is also not impossible that there could be significant attitude shifts in the near future.

The American health care system is not a system: the public sector has shifted somewhat from a federal to a state and local emphasis, and the private sector is alive with diversity and almost unruly experimentation. Although we shall be discussing this in greater depth as we explore the bureaucratic theme in Chapters 5 and 6, it is important to make a major point or two to orient the reader to the overall perspective. For decades, this country has had successful examples of prepaid, comprehensive health programs (such as the Kaiser Health Plan), wherein high quality care is rendered for considerably lower cost, often at the expense of some freedom of choice on the patient's part and generally utilizing a generalist physician in the gatekeeper role who controls access to hospitalization, laboratory tests, and specialists. "Managed care" has become the buzzword these days, meaning cost-effective activity will receive high priority. Always there have been predictions that the HMO or some analogue of an HMO would sweep the nation, driving out the solo private practitioner, but such has never occurred, although there have been modest increases in our national participation in HMOs. In the past few years, however, in some areas there have been dramatic increases in HMO enrollment, reaching the 50 percent level in Minneapolis–St. Paul, for example.

One of the main reasons why this trend may now be on a roll is the unequivocal evidence of a relative surfeit of physicians. That is, well-trained young physicians are more than happy to take a salaried position in a managed care environment because the options are dwindling elsewhere. The frightening malpractice situation, no doubt, is contributing to making an organizational setting relatively more appealing than solo private practice as a practice modality for doctors just starting out. In any case, the number of doctors is increasing steadily and will continue to provide high-caliber professionals to fuel the engines of the prepaid comprehensive care provider organizations as they race toward dominance of what has traditionally been a cottage industry.

Finally, there needs to be an observation made about the overall status of the cost of American health care. Ours is the highest, but that needn't be anything to be ashamed of. If ours is the best health care in the world, then we should be proud of it—and we can be proud of our medical science and of the enormous advances our investment in health has brought to us and the world. We are preeminent still in this field in all the world and we shall undoubtedly lose some of that if we construct an environment in which the brightest young people increasingly elect other fields. We should remember too that our large investment in health, even if in ineffective practices, provides jobs in a service industry and a market for production industries, the income from which flows primarily into the American economy. If we were to reduce our health expenditures tomorrow from 12 percent to 6 percent of the GNP, we would surely decrease the cost and therefore the price of American-made automobiles and other items, providing more money for Americans to spend on other sectors of the economy, but we would be saddled with an enormous unemployment and retraining problem. My point is not to defend useless or ineffective health care or advocate the status quo or expansion of our total investment in health care; rather, I seek to question the often unspoken assumption that reducing expenditures for health is automatically good for the country's financial status. We already spend less of the public treasury on health than all the other leading Western nations; therefore, most of the potential savings or cuts may be in the private sector. Again, let me reiterate my bias here: there is much for us to do to provide better, more appropriate cost-effective health care in the United States, but dramatic economies might not do our society any more good from an economic standpoint than if we cut our expenditures on cosmetics or electronics or any other industry in half. On the other hand, in those industries where prices are set in the international marketplace, it would obviously be useful to American companies to minimize costs for health care provided to their workers.

As a nation, we are not, in my view, upset so much by the

high cost of our health care as we are by the growing awareness that so much of what we do has not been adequately tested. The series of studies by Wennberg has shown that "standard" practice can vary from community to community and that furthermore doctors are sometimes able to alter their behavior once they are made aware that colleagues in another place are less prone to a particular intervention than they are. There is no doubt that our research establishment has invested overwhelmingly in the molecular biology of health and disease, less so in the public health, disease prevention, and health promotion aspects, but painfully inadequately in the studies of efficacy and treatment outcomes. Thus, our basic and applied research machines are churning out new technologies which find their way into practice without adequate evaluation. In fact, we have a dearth of professionals capable of designing and implementing the proper studies; all too few of our medical journals require the statistical detail and experimental design necessary to insure the acquisition of useful data. Thus, all too often we load ourselves down with an expensive and irrelevant technology. Clearly, the routine use of external fetal monitoring in normal pregnancy is a recent and current example; the monitor frequently emits false positive readings, leading to an inappropriate number of unnecessary Cesarean sections. Thus, we have an incomparable opportunity to attack this technology assessment problem in such a way as to dramatically affect excessive costs and to increase the quality of care rendered. The priority and status of this kind of research must go up if we are to succeed; society has to encourage the best young minds to attack these issues. All the analytic methods and tools are present to accomplish the task. The only sad observation that must be made is that too few of our professional and industrial leaders even recognize this as a problem, much less the main problem. We can no longer guarantee that our clinical practices and interventions are the best money can buy, because we haven't spent enough money to adequately test new technologies before proclaiming them to be standard practice. As this fact dawns upon the American public in a thousand different ways, society can be expected to be increasingly strident in its complaints about the excessive costs of the enterprise. A crisis in trust is upon the doctors as on all health professionals, but the loss of confidence is extending or will extend to institutions as well. Wennberg has recently analyzed hospital data in Boston and New Haven; his analysis indicates that costs are twice as high in Boston as in New Haven for the same product and outcome. Such information will ultimately worry the public and suggests that if there is a golden opportunity for reform for the health establishment in the area of technology assessment, there is a crucial need for such activity to move forward with vigor if permanent damage is to be avoided in societal trust in its health care providers and institutions.

4

THE
HIPPOCRATIC
THEME

Life is short,
The art long,
Opportunity fleeting,
Experience fallacious,
Judgment difficult.
—Hippocrates, Aphorisms I (Adams 1972)

The witchdoctor succeeds for the same reason all the
rest of us succeed. Each patient carries his own doc-
tor inside him. They come to us not knowing that
cure. We are at our best when we give the doctor who
resides within each patient a chance to go to work.
—Albert Schweitzer (in Ornstein and
    Sobel 1987: 258)

I swear by Apollo the physician, and Aesculapius,
and Health, and All-heal, and all the gods and god-
desses, that according to my ability and judgment, I
will keep this Oath and this stipulation—to reckon
him who taught me this Art equally dear to me as my
parents, to share my substance with him, and relieve
his necessities if required; to look upon his offspring
in the same footing as my own brothers, and to teach
them this art, if they shall wish to learn it, without
fee or stipulation; and that by precept, lecture, and
every other mode of instruction, I will impart a
knowledge of the Art to my own sons, and those of
my teachers, and to disciples bound by a stipulation

and oath according to the law of medicine, but to none others.

I will follow that system of regimen which, according to my ability and judgment, I consider for the benefit of my patients, and abstain from whatever is deleterious and mischievous. I will give no deadly medicine to any one if asked, nor suggest any such counsel; and in like manner I will not give to a woman a pessary to produce abortion. With purity and with holiness I will pass my life and practice my Art. I will not cut persons laboring under the stone, but will leave this to be done by men who are practitioners of this work.

Into whatever houses I enter, I will go into them for the benefit of the sick, and will abstain from every voluntary act of mischief and corruption; and, further, from the seduction of females or males, of freemen and slaves. Whatever, in connection with my professional practice or not, I see or hear, in the life of men, which ought not to be spoken of abroad, I will not divulge, as reckoning that all such should be kept secret. While I continue to keep this Oath unviolated, may it be granted to me to enjoy life and the practice of the art, respected by all men, in all times! But should I trespass and violate this Oath, may the reverse be my lot!

This ancient oath, which contains so many particulars which most young modern physicians do not believe, remains the bedrock of the commitment made each year by thousands of graduating medical students. Most thoughtful physicians who have reflected on its meaning conclude that the ancient oath remains popular late in the twentieth century precisely because it proclaims a commitment to the best interests of the patient

and to high professional competence, characteristics of a healing profession which we all think was dramatically changed by
Hippocrates. Now we think that Hippocrates did not write the
oath and probably would not have subscribed to much of it
(Richards 1987). Healing up to Hippocrates' time involved talking, praying, and blatant shamanism, and Hippocrates was ve-
hemently against all that. Occasionally, doctors would be hired
to end a life, with or without the patient's consent, but Hippocrates based his healing on a natural philosophy that placed humankind in harmony with nature rather than in control of it; he
based his interventions on observation, practicality, proof, and
the constant self-warning not to do harm to the patient. His science was dedicated firmly to the patient's welfare. The physician
sought honor through doing right by the sick person. No longer
could the physician be hired to poison someone or become a
purposeful agent of death. Hippocrates eschewed words as therapeutic, calling medicine the silent art. His written descriptions
of some of his cases are masterpieces in clinical observation and
deduction. He was in a word the father of scientific medicine.

Pedro Lain Entralgo, the well-known Spanish psychiatrist,
has traced the history of the spoken word in therapy during the
past three millennia (1970). Of course, the blossoming of the
therapy of the word came with Freud. Lain Entralgo points out,
in fact, that Aristotle understood the essentials of psychiatry's
roots and even advocated the therapeutic value of the audiences'
emotional catharsis through attending the tragedies of the the-
ater. He attributes the greater than two thousand–year wait for
the Freudian insights to the severe proscriptions of Hippocrates
and his followers against the use of the word, shamanism, and
cheering speech in the medical model. This is not the place to
attempt a history of psychiatry since Freud, but it is fair to say
that psychoanalysis and psychotherapy by and large have trav-
eled a separate road from mainstream medical practice, with
psychosomatic medicine serving for many years as a somewhat

insecure bridge between the more biochemically oriented mainstream and the softer sciences of Freudian psychiatry.

In the past two decades, however, the revolutionary advances in the neurosciences have brought mind and body, emotion and molecule together in ways that tend to give words a new therapeutic currency. Instead of the handful of neurochemicals known in the 1960s to function in the brain, we now know that our brain is an extraordinary pharmacy, able to modulate a situation with great precision in response to a wide variety of stimuli (Ornstein and Sobel 1987). Clearly, doctoring has become more than deciding which medicine to use to help a patient; the best doctors will work to create an environment in which the patient can allow his or her own therapeutic capacities to work.

Possibly, the well-known placebo effect is the best example of this; fully 30 percent of patients in certain situations will report significant improvement when given something they believe is curative but which in effect is physiologically inert. One well-known cardiologist claims that, if he can meet one of his patients suffering from an acute heart attack at the hospital emergency room and tell him or her that everything is under control and will be all right, then he can dispense with the usual dose of morphine, presumably because the patient's own endorphins have taken over.

The reverse is also true; words can have adverse effects. Words and actions that distress, anger, or upset a seriously ill person can be a negative force in the healing process. Doctors who used to belong to the most mechanistically inclined groups now can envision in molecular terms why one can get better results by establishing and maintaining a trust relationship with one's patients, or why a destroyed and distrustful relationship can contribute to a less than optimal result in addition to a malpractice suit. Scholars like Erik Erikson (1987) who analyze the nature of the therapeutic relationship now have more heed paid to them; body language, nonverbal and verbal communication skills, and interviewing techniques are getting more and more attention from a profession which for too long has been restricted by an unnecessarily narrow biochemical vision and a scientific gestalt that kept it from fully utilizing approaches, the results of which couldn't be adequately explained in molecular terms. Even now, the laying on of hands inherent in the manipulations of osteopaths and chiropractors is in my view sadly undervalued by traditional medicine, both for the direct benefits of muscle relaxation and neuromuscular relief and for the indirect benefits of direct contact with the caring hands of a concerned and competent professional. A tension headache is better cured when muscles are relaxed by a healer's hands rather than by Valium.

America is a less authoritarian place than most other countries. Still, in years past, one did what the doctor ordered and one did it just because the doctor said to. The therapeutic relationship rested on a trust built upon a perception of the doctor's competence and an acceptance that the doctor knew best. Many forces in our society have worked against this aspect of the doctor-patient relationship. Malpractice suits have become more and more prominent, underscoring the fallibility of the doctor, although the suits usually arise out of poor communication on the doctor's part; public education and sophistication about things medical have led patients to have more doubts and ask more questions; health and medical affairs have become important media items such that currently most newspapers across the United States print in featured columns the gist of the most important articles published that day in the leading medical journals, sometimes two or three days before the doctors themselves even receive the journal in the mail.

In the late 1960s, while serving as the medical director of a university hospital, I had an experience with a malpractice suit which taught me a great deal about the nature of the doctor-patient relationship and the variety of perceptions extant in our society about that relationship. A professor in our law school was participating as a research subject in a study of the effects of graded exercise in normal males, a study which was being conducted by a senior cardiologist. After running to exhaustion on the cardiologist's treadmill in the hospital clinic, he took a hot shower in the hospital clinic's shower room and promptly collapsed and died. Fortunately, the cardiologist was right there, resuscitated him promptly, and saw him through an uneventful recovery from his heart attack in the hospital. Shortly thereafter, the lawyer sued the cardiologist and the hospital. Aside from the availability of unnecessarily hot water for a shower and the absence of a warning not to take a hot shower, the law professor was ecstatic with his cardiologist and the hospital care he received and was adamant in wishing to continue in their care. The patient understood that he unknowingly had been very close to having a heart attack at the time of his study and, in fact, that he was fortunate to have had it in a controlled environment with medical care so close at hand.

His doctor no longer wanted to care for him but the patient insisted, telling me at one point that he saw no reason why a little lawsuit should threaten his relationship with or the mindset of his physician. The lawyer patient did not perceive that an adversarial relationship established by a lawsuit was incompatible with the trust essential for a therapeutic relationship, at least from the physician's point of view. The patient was greatly disappointed when I wrote informing him that we would not care for him at our hospital as long as comparable care was available in the city, with the exception, of course, of emergency care requirements. If this episode clearly illustrates the intrinsic conflict between the adversarial relationship fostered by a lawsuit and the therapeutic relationship, another personal experience illustrates an equally important value conflict between the political or bureaucratic gestalt and that of the average American doctor.

A few years ago, I participated in a symposium including several twenty-fifth reunion classmates at my college. We were each to summarize briefly the quintessential values central to our occupations. I happened to lead off and indicated that what had remained central to my profession was the commitment to the primacy of the individual patient's welfare, such that by oath I was obliged to seek the best available care for my patients, even if that care might be something that as a citizen I would advocate not making available to patients similar to mine. I pointed out that the belief of the patient in the depth of the physician's commitment to what is best for the patient is essential for the sustenance of the trust relationship so important for optimal healing.

Using as an example chronic renal dialysis, I pointed out that patients should be able to count on their physicians to present that therapeutic option to the patients at the appropriate time, whether or not the physician as citizen agrees with a national policy to make that technology available to everyone of every age. If a doctor cannot advocate an available technology or present it as a viable possibility because of a philosophic or religious belief on the doctor's part, such should be made known to the patient and the advisability should be explored of getting another physician better able to serve the patient's best interests according to the patient's perspective.

Toward the end of the line of panelists was a good friend of mine who held one of the most important health policy–making posts in America; to my surprise and chagrin, he launched a spirited attack on what I had said. In essence, he indicated my stated views encapsulated all that was bad and irresponsible about medical doctors, that since doctors directly or indirectly were responsible for 70 percent of health care costs they should be willing to make rationing decisions and thereby help solve the cost crisis in health care. In my view, this bureaucratic perception of the doctor as rationer is as destructive as the adversarial stance of the malpractice lawyer to the capacity to have in full bloom the much-sought-after therapeutic relationship.

In the early 1960s the doctrine of informed consent swept into American medicine through the clinical research window but has had since then a far-reaching effect on the day-to-day practice of medicine, where patients are required to sign documents that indicate that they have had full explanations of all the details of side effects and the costs and benefits of a proposed intervention before such is undertaken.

The American courts have reached into the medical record, exposing every detail to public scrutiny in nasty malpractice cases; increasingly over the past decade there have emerged serious proponents of giving patients their own medical records, an approach which certainly requires a tactful but honest write-up by the doctor. Influential physicians began to advocate telling the cold truth to all patients about their condition, albeit they might advocate telling them in a humane and warmly sensitive way. Advocates of this approach point to the growing literature from dying patients, a literature which describes the isolation and degradation of the terminal patient, made all the worse by the doctor's denial of the truth. There are many examples of dramatic alterations in patient behavior after having someone tell them the truth; the American patient dying of cancer will generally prefer a doctor who will tell him or her the truth and stick with him or her through thick or thin until the end over a doctor who adopts a falsely cheerful attitude, never speaking about the disease or the likely outcome and distancing him- or herself emotionally from the real situation of the patient. The belief has grown in American medicine that this candor about death, once so seldom practiced, has allowed death with dignity to become more standard.

Candor and truthfulness have spilled over into all elements of the doctor-patient relationship to the extent that Sissela Bok

(1979) believes that giving placebos is dishonest, deceitful, and ultimately destructive to the patient and to medicine. Although not everyone fully accepts Bok's rather purist approach to these points, most people now believe that candor, honesty, full disclosure, and openness on the part of the physician form the basis of that special trust which is central to the formation of the desired therapeutic relationship.

With unquestioned physician authority essentially a thing of the past, clearly and continually demonstrated integrity is required. The authoritarian nature of the doctor-patient relationship has so diminished as an operative mode in America that a popular newswriter recently referred to her new doctor as George Smith, J.P., where the J.P. stands for junior partner. Her doctor presents her with options, information, decision trees, statistical probabilities, and side effects of proposed medications, ranging along a continuum from "relatively benign" to "downright terrifying." Her J.P. also teaches her how to live "healthfully."

Although there is obviously great overlapping of values shared by the American and British medical professions, this matter of informed consent may be a key difference between them. In America, largely as a result of the informed consent movement and court opinions, the pendulum has swung from the doctor to the patient as the decision maker. Repeatedly, the courts have punished doctors in malpractice decisions for not recognizing that the patient is in charge and in fact needs to be made aware of all the known salient details about his own case. The argument for "informed consent" in America rests on the "liberty interests" of the individual as defined only twenty-five years ago by our judiciary, making it a complex matter to reverse this new American tilt toward the patient as captain of the ship (Katz 1984). The Supreme Court has decided that in fact the medical record belongs to the patient. In Britain, on the other hand, the Sidaway case in December 1984 produced a decision that left the doctor essentially in charge of the information flow to the patient; in England the doctor is still firmly in command, required to tell the patient no more than is customary.

A further ramification of the informed consent movement in the United States was indicated by Charles Begley (1987), an American health economist, who concluded in a recent essay that "a prospective payment system that asked physicians to allocate limited resources may not be able to tolerate the patient-oriented doctrine of informed consent." Certainly, the National Health Service is essentially a prospective payment system; if Begley is correct, one might expect that, should an American-size informed consent movement strike England, there will emerge increasing conflict in the system.

In Russia recently an American physician helped resuscitate a patient who subsequently asked the Russian-speaking American what had happened. When the American told the Russian, the latter seemed greatly relieved, but the American was called on the carpet by a Soviet colleague who pointed out that in Russia they never told patients that sort of thing, that they didn't believe the patients could tolerate it, and the American learned that different cultures handle things differently.

A German oncologist, trained at some of America's leading institutions, recently elaborated on this phenomenon in a conversation with me. When he went to America as a young physician for specialty training, he was used to the traditional, old-school authoritarian approach by the doctor to the patient. In America over four years he learned from his mentors to be more open and communicative with his patients. Then, he returned to a leading medical center in Germany and for two years persisted in his more open approach, despite the fact that he confused the patients and often his colleagues. This approach finally caused him enough grief with the patients and the doctors referring them to him that he reluctantly abandoned it. He said that, quite simply, the German patient didn't like or want anything other than the paternalistic, more authoritarian manner and that the

German doctor could be more effective by using it, at least for the time being.

Although it may be stretching the point, the informed consent movement seems connected to the move to recapture citizen competence, to reassert the individual's responsibility for his or her own health and welfare, and to emphasize that the next great advances in the improvement of the health status of the American people would be made through education and behavior modification. Although these efforts at health promotion and disease prevention are society-wide, it is clear that the family or primary physician is a very important player. More and more doctors, previously disease and treatment oriented, appreciate these days that some of their most effective contributions come in the prevention areas.

The whole nation takes pride in our improving statistics in cancer, cardiac disease, stroke, and hypertension. We know that, with the exception of lung cancer, the reasons for the advances are not clear. We believe in general, however, that the movement to individual responsibility for one's own health is important. In my view, this movement is not unconnected with the informed consent movement and the general effort to demythologize the physician and reduce his or her power and influence. Regardless of other perhaps less beneficial outcomes of informed consent, this outcome must be recognized as highly positive.

For many years, anthropologists have documented the significance of cultural differences in the perceptions of diseases and therapies and even in what precisely distinguishes the concepts of illness and disease. Studies such as those of Tancredi and Romanucci-Ross (1987) and Majno (1987) and the significant work of Kleinman (1980) have reflected and uncovered important elements in the process of healing. As Dr. Guido Majno has pointed out, the important elements of the native American medicine man's healing of a patient grow out of the extraordinary attention paid to the sufferer (many people joining in a ceremony that lasts several days), the ritual itself, and the bringing together of family and community to join in focusing on the improvement of the sick person. Under such conditions, it's easy to imagine that in some or even many instances, curative or ameliorative juices would begin to flow, that immunologic competence might return to a disabled system, and so on. When one considers that the modern hospital is itself a cultural phenomenon, a symbol of healing for most people, one cannot help worrying about the impact of the changing hospital environment on the healing context. Through anthropology, the society and the profession have just begun to learn a great deal more about the perception and interpretation of illness, lessons that are underscored by the rapidly expanding cultural diversity being thrust upon our country by the significant immigrations from Central and South America and Southeast Asia.

Twenty-five years ago I knew of a patient who had had a spontaneous remission of metastatic carcinoma of the lung which seemed to follow an angry outburst from the patient to the doctor (who had diagnosed the problem and suggested that the patient should get his affairs in order); in today's terms the patient's anger may have enhanced his immunologic competence. Although challenged by at least one study recently, there remains a clinical belief that patients who get angry at their disease, at least when that disease is cancer, tend to live longer. Trust, honesty, anger . . . ? How do we put all this together? The only things certain are that often emotions can positively affect outcome and that much research needs to be done on these matters in the years ahead. The studies by bona fide physiologists like Dr. Herbert Benson on people at prayer and on Eastern mystics as they melt the snow around them by redirecting their blood flow to the periphery have all contributed to the current stage wherein modern scientific medicine sits poised to absorb holistic medicine and approaches previously assumed to be at the fringe or beyond.

But technology intrudes once more. If the introduction of the stethoscope established a tool that symbolically stood between patient and doctor, the ever strengthening technological imperative in medicine with computers, laboratory profiles, nuclear magnetic resonance, and positron emission tomography could serve to eliminate all human qualities indigenous to the relationship between patient and technocrat-physician-engineer. But should it? Stanley Reiser, the well-known historian of medicine, answers in the negative (Reiser and Anbar 1984). In his view, the computer and the other spectacular advances should provide adequate time for mature physicians to more thoroughly talk and interact with their patients. One could argue that, instead of consigning the modern American physician to the healer's junk pile, we might postulate the dawning of a new era for the scientific healer.

Having provided the doctor, the official high priest of technology in the service of humankind, with the most spectacular new tools, one can also offer a deepening understanding of the values, techniques, and results of making successful therapeutic relationships. Physician time must be valued, just as is technical skill. By maintaining integrity, compassion, and competence in our commitment to the patient and by deepening our understanding of the therapeutic relationship, a new modern Hippocrates could be in the making, a healer with hitherto unimagined powers. A modern Hippocratic Oath might read as follows:

The Oath of the Modern Hippocrates, 1988

By all that I hold highest, I promise my patients competence, integrity, candor, personal commitment to their best interests, compassion, and absolute discretion and confidentiality within the law.
I shall do by my patients as I would be done by, shall obtain consultation whenever I or they desire, shall educate them

and include them to the extent they wish in all important decisions, and shall minimize suffering whenever a cure cannot be obtained, understanding that a dignified death is an important goal in everyone's life.

I shall try to establish a friendly relationship with my patients and shall accept each one in a nonjudgmental manner, appreciating the validity and worth of different value systems and according to each person a full measure of human dignity.

I shall charge only for my professional services and shall not profit financially in any other way as a result of the advice and care I render my patients.

I shall provide advice and encouragement for my patients in their efforts to sustain their own health.

I shall work with my profession to improve the quality of medical care and to improve the public health. As a citizen, I shall work for equitable health care for all, but I shall not let other public or professional considerations however important interfere with my primary commitment to provide the best and most appropriate care available to each of my patients.

To the extent that I live by these precepts, I shall be a worthy physician.

In summary, without regard for organization and finances and considering strictly the history of the Hippocratic theme and the incredible scientific achievements of the past fifty years, the following can be stated about American health care:

1. We have the most powerful curative and preventive interventions in our history.
2. We have a medical profession populated in abundance with well-educated, talented people and generally united in a commitment to human service and high competence.
3. We have an array of over one hundred academic health

science centers each with a variety of health professional schools and associated teaching hospitals.

4. We have well-prepared and dedicated researchers who are on the brink of even more astounding technological and scientific breakthroughs in the understanding and amelioration of diseases.

5. We have a new appreciation of speech and affect as therapeutic, opening the way to a greater incorporation and amalgamation of the "holistic" alternative approaches with the scientific.

6. We have a public that still trusts its doctors, dentists, and nurses.

7. When all these things are taken together, we have the prospect of the development of the greatest cadre of healers the world has known. The need, if all this is true, is for broader, not narrower, education and a greater, not lesser, sense of the wholeness of the human being, of the wholeness of intellectual effort, and the connectedness of the sciences and the arts.

The procompetitive health care scene in America seems to threaten many thoughtful leaders. Why does it so threaten these professionals? It is the threat to the core of physicianhood as expressed in the Hippocratic theme that drives these concerns and anxieties. The core of modern physicianhood doesn't rest in a payment mechanism, an organizational model, or a practice paradigm; it rests in the vision, the operative ideal that emerges when the central ideals of Hippocrates are intertwined with the driving force of modern science. It is this vision or operative ideal that many policy makers have neglected, that critics have failed to consider adequately, and that doctors everywhere fear losing by strategies aimed at profits and efficiencies. For such doctors, destroying the Hippocratic tradition will be throwing the baby out with the bathwater; it will be organizing and competing ourselves out of a profession of scientifically based healers.

Let us now turn to the bureaucratic imperative which has recently produced such dramatic changes and explore the potential conflicts and synergies between the two themes.

5 THE BUREAUCRATIC THEME

Most of us realize that an accurate history cannot be recorded by an active participant immersed in the unfolding events he or she seeks to describe, but it remains a lesson we consistently overlook. We are swept away by the pace of change, by our need to anticipate it; we have given birth to a whole new cadre of "futurists," many of whom have no credentials sufficient to elicit our trust in their insight or perspicacity but who may well have access to a printing press or a television camera. Most educated people, then, understand that journalists cannot write an accurate or complete history and appreciate equally well the many examples within recent memory of trends which according to the best experts seemed certain to yield predictable results but which somehow did not end up that way after all; and yet we all too readily tend to accept as inevitable a future condition that in reality may still be amenable to change. In so doing we yield our birthright to citizenship in a democratic society; we give up the potential in such instances for competent citizenship, for working in responsible ways to shape a future consistent with our most basic values. Almost no one wants to tilt at windmills all day long, because a life of practical futility, however noble or saintly, has little appeal in the modern utilitarian world. On the other hand, some windmills might in fact not yet be firmly anchored on their foundations and might therefore be amenable to being knocked over. This judgment about which windmills to select for what may seem a quixotic charge is one of the most difficult yet most important and potentially creative decisions to be made by people active in the health policy area.

The current debate in the United States is full of good examples of important health policy players choosing windmills with which to tilt, largely because health care in America is clearly in a state of rapid and dramatic transition. Some people seem certain of their foreknowledge of the steady-state condition that will obtain when this current process of the deregulation of the health care industry runs its course. While many experts accept the inevitable drift toward a new procompetitive state and are devising strategies for optimal survival and functioning under those conditions, others foresee no good to come of it, predict a loss of the essential value-based nature of the health enterprise, and advocate a rapid alteration in course.

It is my purpose here to offer my own account of the current state of American health care, leading to some interpretive comments and ideally the development of the most pertinent questions for a competent citizenry to ask in the years ahead. This "history" is not and cannot be complete; it will be painted with broad strokes and will focus more intently upon matters which relate to the value questions we've chosen to explore here. To begin, let me express a few assumptions and biases.

First, everything I have seen supports the view of Professor Don Price that policy making in America can best be thought of as "creeping incrementalism." The United Kingdom seemed to reach a decision after World War II that truly equal access to health care for its population was the right thing. A report emerged which made great good sense, had enormous prestige, and received wide attention and national debate. Adjustments were made to the plan in a timely fashion and the dramatic innovation of the National Health Service was implemented. The successes of that system's widespread implementation in the United Kingdom are well known to all. The process of planning and implementation of the National Health Service clearly is not an example of creeping incrementalism.

Creeping incrementalism is passing an amendment in 1972 to the American Social Security Act allowing Medicare (previously restricted to health care for the elderly) to cover chronic kidney dialysis for people of all ages without any serious public debate or analysis of impact. Creeping incrementalism is having the United States government pay medical schools large sums of money to increase their enrollment, while Joseph Califano, as the cabinet officer responsible for the program, publicly castigates medical education leaders for irresponsibility in flooding the market with new doctors. Thus, creeping incrementalism can be thought of as that political doctrine which allows a nation to move from drastic underproduction to dramatic overproduction of physicians in a step-by-step manner without ever having achieved a level of production that was identified as proper!

The second assumption is that special interest groups in the United States play an enormous role in the way policy is made and expressed through the federal budget. This assumption addresses the fact that the defense establishment competes with the health establishment, the education establishment, the research and technology development establishment, the transportation establishment, etc. for a proper-sized piece of the federal pie.

My third general bias is that Calabresi and Bobbitt's (1978) conceptualization of societal tragic choices more accurately describes than any other paradigm what goes on in a Western-style democracy in the process of making choices (which we refer to euphemistically as "policy making"). In brief, it is their view that every societal choice leaves someone out, even consigning them to death; in time, since society cannot tolerate this, a shift in values must occur to favor in some way those who suffered under the previous policy. The tragedy in a way is spread around without ever having to publicly admit that we commit some to death. A good example is the military draft guidelines, which tend to exempt from service certain people.

The fourth general bias relates to the inappropriateness of assuming that the United States is the quintessential mass culture made up of a homogeneous army of television-shaped teeny-boppers or ex-teenyboppers whose values are shared in all-important details in every quarter of the nation. A simple overlay superimposition of the land mass of the United States on that of western Europe reveals that over twenty European nations would fit within the borders of the continental United States. In biology, we used to argue whether form followed function or whether form determined function; it seems to me that the physical characteristics of America, its size and diversity, are an important influence on the creeping incrementalism of our national policy development. A democracy, particularly a large and diverse one, expresses many values through its national policies; national policies make choices that favor some people and their values and may detract from others; hence, Calabresi's term *tragic choices* and his view that fairness in a democratic society requires a periodic shifting to address the interests of those whose lives and values have not been emphasized under current policies. So the pendulum swings, destined only to move again in yet another direction so as to allow the entire nation to persist in the myth that it is not sacrificing some people with each deci-. sion. For America, then, tragic choices and creeping incremen-talism are all of a piece and are likely to be characteristic of our policy making as long as we survive as a democratic state. But that doesn't mean that a coherent story cannot unfold. Let us turn to the health policy story of the United States over the past four decades.

Looked at from a policy perspective, national health policy in the post–World War II period has been an unqualified success. Although the times and climate favored the fullest flowering of the great American problem-solving technique (i.e., once the problem has been carefully identified, throw large amounts of money at it and eventually it will be solved), there is much of which our nation can be proud. What was evolving during the fifties and early sixties was the concept of all citizens' right to health care of the highest order. The federal government was on a roll; Uncle Sam would deal with all important matters.

It was determined that our hospitals were old and dilapidated and contained too few beds. A law was passed, money was budgeted, and, within a decade or so, we had lots of modern hospital beds.

We needed more science and technology for the benefit of the public. Therefore, disease by disease, we attacked the research and specialty care needs of our nation; Jim Shannon, director of NIH, Senator Lister Hill of Alabama, and Congressman Fogarty of Rhode Island led a small group of influential leaders in the successful fight to increase the nation's spending on biomedical research. We trained specialists and researchers, thus enlarging our medical school faculties by sixfold over the past fifteen or twenty years.

We perceived a severe doctor shortage. Congress passed a law and the number of medical school graduates increased from seven thousand in 1967 to sixteen thousand in 1985.

We perceived a need for more specialists. We passed a law to support specialty training. We perceived a need for more primary care doctors, so Congress appropriated the requisite dollars to stimulate the growth of family practice residencies.

We perceived a need for broader accessibility to health care for all sectors of our society. We developed Medicare and Medicaid, gave tax credits to employers who provided health insurance for their workers, and elevated the proportion of our population with health insurance to greater than 85 percent. Over the past ten years, minorities and the poor have clearly improved their access to health care, visiting the doctor each year as often as the average white client and, in many states, achieving equal access to all hospitals. In other words, great strides were made toward the achievement of a single class of care for all.

In all of these changes, the profession of medicine through its primary organization, the American Medical Association (AMA), fought to preserve what it perceived to be the best interests of the doctor. In the late forties and early fifties, the AMA successfully fought off the U.S. government in all major health initiatives. As pointed out by Wilbur Cohen, the passage in 1965 of the Social Security legislation establishing Medicare demonstrated for the first time that the power of the AMA could be broken, and it has been diminishing more or less ever since.

The one area in which the AMA has retained its success rate in the policy arena has been in the maintenance of the fee-for-service system of payment for physicians. As the financing system evolved in both the public and private sectors, the physician always received "reasonable and customary" fees. Until the widespread advent of health insurance, both public and private, there was a proud and important tradition among physicians wherein they freely devoted their services to people who couldn't pay and equally generously gave their time to educate medical students and residents. The so-called Robin Hood syndrome occurred in which the well-to-do supported physicians and those efforts they were able and willing to give away.

Within a decade, that tradition of contributing free care and free teaching dissolved. Payment was received through third-party insurers (including Medicare and Medicaid) who paid for whatever the physician did according to "usual and customary" standards. Now, therefore, the third-party payers were paying physicians at rates that previously had allowed them to carry on like Robin Hood, except that the Medicare and Medicaid programs provided reimbursement for the elderly and poor, assisting the trend to some dramatic income increases for many physicians. Increasingly, teaching physicians learned how to bill for their services while teaching, again especially for the poor. A significant characteristic of much of medical practice was disappearing too, and that was the direct payment of the physician by the patient for personal services rendered. Though the loss of this way of transacting business was fought by the profession, and very sincerely so, the rapid expansion of physician incomes and the obvious enhancement of accessibility to health care for those previously unable to pay rendered this opposition ultimately insignificant. This same trend toward cross-subsidization of care for the poor and for teaching costs occurred with hospitals, and almost imperceptibly these two major efforts were loaded onto the cart being pulled by the private insurers on behalf of employers.

In the 1930s, at the Rip Van Winkle Clinic in New York state, a successful prepaid program was established wherein for a flat fee all necessary health care would be provided to participants. This was the first Health Maintenance Organization (HMO). During World War II, Henry J. Kaiser provided a system of total health care for his workers which evolved in the postwar era to include a growing number of subscribers, largely in Hawaii and the West Coast of the United States. Other similar institutions sprang up here and there and flourished in modest ways through the 1960s and 1970s; the HMO effort was a crusade for some and was strongly advocated by many experts, but it experienced great difficulty in getting widespread national acceptance. Far less than 10 percent of the population was ever enrolled in these health care plans prior to the past few years. Most doctors preferred the solo practice of medicine or group practices which generally allowed for more independence, were more professionally satisfying, and were usually more lucrative than employment in an HMO. Organized medicine and other elements of society actively opposed the flourishing of HMOs. It was not uncommon for people to be HMO members until they got really sick and then they would go outside the HMO to get the level of expertise they wanted or thought they needed.

Health care benefits became an important item in labor relations as labor-management contracts, which provided health care as an increasingly major fringe benefit for large numbers of workers, were negotiated. Complete health insurance is a wonderful fringe benefit, because it is of potentially great financial value should serious illness strike the individual. It was very appealing for both labor and management to negotiate; therefore, there was a rapid expansion of private insurance programs available to the working population and to their families. For reasons that have always been obscure to me but must obviously have been related to financial performance, the insurance carriers persisted in covering in-hospital care more readily than out-of-hospital care. They also paid more for procedures or laboratory tests than they did for the doctor's time. Thus, the patient would typically have to pay from his or her own pocket for a diagnostic evaluation done in the out-patient clinic, whereas if hospitalized the insurance company would cover all expenses. Further, the doctor would frequently find that his patient or the patient's family would prefer to have the patient stay in the hospital for continuing therapies or rehabilitative services which could have been provided on an out-patient basis. Such a course of extended hospitalization seemed to hurt no one and often on the surface seemed to help everyone, impacting only on the insurance premium, which was of course spread across a large, impersonal, and unaware group.

This approach to paying hospitals and doctors obviously encouraged the provision of more services, doing more procedures and more tests, because in general they seemed to be "free" to the patient. There were other results from this kind of approach. For example, as malpractice suits began to increase, doctors found it easier to practice "defensive" medicine, ordering tests that were largely unnecessary for diagnosis but that might come in handy in case the doctors were sued. Another example is the incentive this reimbursement mechanism provided to physicians to become adept at certain procedures which were reimbursable in the ambulatory setting to make up for income not forthcoming for the time that the doctor might spend talking with the patient.

As one might have guessed, in addition to increased accessibility to effective health care for our citizenry, the net result of all these policies has been a steady annual growth in health care costs and expenditures. Along with these signs of success, there naturally came the detractors or the advocates of the other side of the coin. For the detractors, the costs were too high; hospitals were over-bedded and therefore must not be running efficiently; doctors' incomes were growing rapidly and their conspicuous consumption was annoying; pharmaceutical companies were seen to be controlling our lives, encouraging us through advertising to become a pill-taking society and thereby profiting from our weaknesses; new technologies and drugs were being utilized on patients too soon and without adequate testing. As the proportion of the health care dollar that was paid by the government increased, the federal dollars available to other significant constituents diminished and, pretty soon, the health care dollar became a worthy target for competing constituencies.

Due to this, federal attempts to regulate and control health care costs grew and each of these governmental efforts was seen as an intrusion by the basically politically conservative profession of medicine, which therefore resisted them. The forces for centralized governmental approaches gathered strength and we saw a wide variety of regulatory and planning efforts flow from the Johnson, Nixon, and Carter administrations. In some states, hospital charges were strictly regulated by state agencies. Highly intrusive innovations labeled "quality assurance mechanisms" were widely implemented, even though these massive governmentally sponsored efforts were really aimed at cost control rather than quality enhancement. In spite of this, there was little demonstrable effect upon the ever-escalating costs of health care.

I remember clearly an informal meeting in 1973 in Washington, D.C. at which a distinguished British physician listened to a description of the new Professional Services Review Organizations that the U.S. government was putting into place. His response was one of amazement, because he said the National Health Service would never agree to intrude to such an incredible extent on the independent authority of the physician to practice medicine.

Important societal voices (in addition to those of the detractors discussed above) began to be raised in opposition to these increasing costs, to the domination of high technology in health care, and to the seemingly unlimited authority of the physician. Critics aimed to demythologize the physician and the so-called medical model through which, it was claimed, the profession had for years maintained its stranglehold on health policy and health care. Such critics pointed out that relatively large proportions of patients entering the hospital acquired other, sometimes lethal, diseases while there. Epidemiologists poked holes in long-established treatment modalities, showing in one famous situation that a sham open heart operation produced results at least as positive as did the operative intervention then in vogue to increase coronary artery blood flow. Archie Cochrane, the well-known British epidemiologist, was for a time in the mid-seventies an extremely influential force in policy circles in Washington, D.C. He frequently referred to a published British study which showed that those people who received treatment at home for an acute myocardial infarction did better than those who went into the coronary care unit in the hospital. This came at a time when U.S. hospitals had just gone into competition with each other to put in place, at great expense, the highly expensive coronary care unit. The British study, as well as Dr. Cochrane's appealing personal presentation of the data, did much at that time to cast doubt in the mind of the federal bureaucracy about the unqualified success of high technology and underscored the growing belief that cost control was too big to be left solely to the judgment of the physician, who directly or indirectly controlled 70 percent of the total health care bill. That Dr.

Cochrane's results could not fairly be transposed with such certainty to the United States made no matter to the impact on federal policy makers.

At this point, my history must be interrupted for a discussion of a movement in the American polity which at first seemed completely unrelated to health care but which was gaining strength and momentum. When the windmills, at which this movement aimed, actually were toppled, it became clear that analogous efforts might succeed in health care. I refer to the process of deregulation of a series of American industries, thought of since the 1930s as quasi-public utilities requiring oversight by specially created, specific federal agencies to protect the public interest. Martha Derthick and Paul Quirk, in their recent book *The Politics of Deregulation* (1985), have made a convincing argument that, contrary to popular belief, the successful deregulation of the trucking, airline, and telecommunications industries represented a victory of rational analysis by expert economists acting in concert with the regulatory agencies and the Congress to overcome the powerful special interest coalitions represented by the corporations and unions, which profited for so long through the regulatory arrangements. The steps taken in each of these three instances of dramatic executions of the sacred cows of government regulation are matters of public record in the 1970s and early 1980s. The outcomes from the public's perspective, and even to some extent from the business community's, have been laudatory, more positive perhaps than most people expected. The changes were accomplished quite rapidly, are working to people's benefit, and seem irreversible for the foreseeable future. In each instance, competition in the marketplace was encouraged, government control and influence were minimized, the power of the unions was diminished, and new wage schedules were established to meet price competition. Procompetition economists and lawyers like Alain Enthoven and Clark Havighurst argued that the same thing could and should be done for health care, a service industry which should be placed in the marketplace like everything else.

By 1980, when Ronald Reagan swept into power, the scene was set for dramatic change in the health care arena. The profession of medicine generally supported the business-oriented, deregulation approach espoused by Reagan, his commitment to the reduction of government power and its capacity to interfere with market forces. He was, by and large, the doctors' cup of tea! The airline, trucking, and telecommunications industries had been deregulated or were close to that condition; but, piece by piece, under Reagan and the Congress, so has the health care industry also been deregulated. In the process, organized medicine appears to have lost forever its ability to preserve the fee-for-service system as the dominant force in physician payment. In successfully holding off Big Brother in the form of Uncle Sam as the major employer of physicians, America seems ready to substitute corporations as major employers of physicians as part of total health care delivery packages for large segments of the population. Joining forces with the Reagan government in its approach to cost control was a powerful new ally in the form of the business coalitions of corporations seeking to improve the market success and sophistication of the aggregate purchaser of health care and committed to reducing the costs of providing health care for their employees. Unions were losing credibility and clout; the president's trouncing of the air controllers' union in his first term proved that point. The fact that over $500 in health care costs went into every new car meant that health care got partially blamed for the loss by America of world preeminence in automobile sales to the Japanese. For the first time, businesses decided to become prudent aggregate buyers of health care and new initiatives to cut costs came into being.

The most striking personifications of these changes are represented by Lee Iacocca, Donald Fraser, and Joseph Califano. In the fifties and sixties, they represented industry, labor unions, and government, respectively, in seeking to increase access to health care, advocating the individual's basic right to health care, and promoting centralized planning and a regulatory apparatus to control costs of health care. Now they all serve on the Chrysler Corporation Board, linked in their effort to reduce the company's costs, attempting to eliminate cross-subsidization so that no Chrysler health care dollars go either to care for the poor or for the education of future doctors.

For-profit hospital chains attracted attention and have had such a meteoric rise into the national consciousness that the Institute of Medicine (IOM) of the National Academy of Sciences conducted a major study of the impact of for-profit chains on American health care. Completed in 1986, this study showed that for-profit chains were neither more efficient nor less effective in delivering care than their not-for-profit counterparts and often provided their stockholders with profits to an amount equal to an excess of charges over those levied by their not-for-profit counterparts. Further, the IOM study showed that the rise in the number of hospitals and beds owned by for-profit chains came largely as a result of their acquisition of so-called proprietary hospitals (i.e., hospitals which were previously owned by individuals on a for-profit basis); the acquisitions usually resulted in an upgrading of the facility and an increase in quality over that produced by the often local (frequently physician) ownership.

Finally, the enormous success enjoyed over a relatively brief period on the stock market by the more successful of these companies disappeared when it became evident that these profits occurred only because of their adroit manipulation of the old system of reimbursement, which had been standard through 1983.

When the government changed in 1984 to payment of hospitals according to a diagnosis-related preset formula, the incentives changed to favor care provided with a minimum of laboratory tests, procedures, and consultations. Thus, if a hospital could take care of a patient for x dollars less than the formula designated for that disease, then the hospital could realize x dollars of profit. Under these new conditions, the for-profit chains lost their edge. They had failed to appreciate the need to switch to out-of-hospital care to make a profit in the new order and they were left holding the bag; the doctors stood to profit just as handsomely from caring for people out of the hospital. Suddenly, the incentives were reversed and behavior was changed; the ill-prepared for-profit chains have been suffering and it seems highly unlikely that they will dominate the industry. Average length of stay in the hospital has dropped by as much as four days per stay in some instances; out-patient surgeries have emerged; and one can foresee the day when the hospital will be essentially a large intensive care unit.

The HMOs are ideally placed to take advantage of this new situation. In Minneapolis/St. Paul, where HMOs now have greater than 50 percent of the market, much of interest is being learned. For example, subscribers will change HMOs if they can save $15 a month; they will change for more convenient or more courteous service; and they assume that there is high quality medical professional care in each situation until they experience or become convinced otherwise.

HMOs deliver a full range of health care to a population by reversing the trend in America from increasing numbers of specialists to more family or general physicians. They also employ the primary physician in a gatekeeper role much as occurs in the NHS, except that HMOs tend to be large group practices wherein primary care doctors share offices and resources with specialists; therefore, these gatekeepers tend to concur with specialists about the proper time for referral.

The large aggregate purchaser of health care has become highly sophisticated and is generally seeking a contractual arrangement that will guarantee a lower cost but preserve quality. To provide these elements requires health facilities, both in-hospital and out, financial support, and good doctors. In the past, it was the doctor who was in short supply; now, thanks to the so-called surplus of well-educated young physicians, there are plenty of talented people willing to work for a salary in order to be able to practice at all. The revolution in health care delivery is thus being fueled by the increased size of the physician pool, and it is this fact that at least in part explains the ambiguity in health policy circles about the need or value of reducing medical school class sizes.

While some people are seeking a return to past conditions, others like Paul Ellwood predict a sweeping change, with the great majority of health care in the United States by the year 2000 being delivered by health care corporations of various sorts. Ellwood has postulated that there may be ten or twenty megacorporations providing health care nationally backed up by a larger number of regionally based smaller companies. If they employ the gatekeeper concept, the health care dollar will shift dramatically from the hospital and the specialist to the outpatient clinic and the generalist and overall costs will go down. While his earlier predictions may be extreme, the trend is still going in his direction. Whether for-profit or not-for-profit, the vertically integrated corporations' domination of health care in the United States is a distinct possibility. How these changes will get implemented and how they will impact upon the Hippocratic tradition is unknown. These and other questions will be considered in the final chapter, after a more detailed discussion of allocating scarce resources or rationing.

Organized medicine appears deeply disappointed. After fighting so valiantly against the forces advocating increasing government control, which remained in the ascendancy throughout the sixties and seventies, it helped to elect the anti–big government forces of the Reagan administration. At last, no more health planning or regulation; no more give-away programs providing all patients with the potential to receive care anywhere; no more

Professional Services Review Organizations health planning agencies, or National Health Service Corps, no chance of Uncle Sam becoming the doctor's employer!

Alas, it is now dawning on the AMA that it has been hoisted with its own petard. Health care became less regulated, all right. The enterprise got treated as a business. The Federal Trade Commission refused to allow any discussion of proper fees and banned the ban on physician advertising. The government reversed financial incentives in order to discourage hospital care; it took steps to open hospital staffs to more physicians and other personnel; it struck down barriers to HMO development; and it has done nothing significant to stem the tide of foreign medical graduates swelling physician ranks and has thus not implemented a policy favoring a diminished output of new physicians. Financial incentives and budget cuts have made for a fiercely competitive business environment as doctors' groups, hospitals, and other companies fight over the population for market share, sometimes with advertisements that would make an automobile salesman blush. There is even a for-profit clinical research company in Tennessee.

Gradually, it is dawning on medicine's leaders that doctors are in danger not of employment by Uncle Sam but of employment by any one of a number of health care companies. The companies can be expected to pay as little as possible to attract the necessary talent and might discharge those doctors who make trouble, who do not see patients rapidly enough, or who are too noisy in their patient advocacy. Many are convinced that, what previous presidents couldn't do in twenty years of treating health care as a right (i.e., control expenditures through top-down regulation), this president has accomplished in seven years of enhanced competition, even though it is now clear that health care is no longer considered a "right." Despite the news that last year health care costs rose seven times more rapidly than the consumer price index, supporters of the procompetitive approach remain optimistic about its ability to control runaway costs.

Health care has become a business and it has become a mélange of big businesses; solo or small businesspersons are on their way out. Thus, the rules of big business will govern the enterprise increasingly. The manager will become more powerful than the doctor; market-sensitive practices will guide the behavior of the group; price and profits will become major considerations; wholesale deals and cut rates will become commonplace as negotiated contracts increasingly govern daily practices; advertising, loss leaders, market shares, and interest in consortia or related businesses will dominate the rhetoric and context of the business. A characteristic model might be that of a for-profit hospital chain buying an insurance company to provide expertise and financing for large population health care; the new conglomerate would then hire doctors, build medical office buildings, and acquire nursing homes, psychiatric hospitals, pharmacies, and hospital supply companies. This is called vertical integration and will occur just as readily with not-for-profit chains. The conglomerate is so big that it might as well be the government from the perspective of the individual physician.

Without regard for the implications of the Hippocratic theme and considering only the bureaucratic theme, one could summarize our position in 1988 as follows:

1. A modest success in turning the tide of rising hospital costs, although total health costs continue to rise presumably because of cost shifting to nonhospital sectors.
2. The creation of fiscal incentives to do less rather than more.
3. The thrust to out-patient care and group practice—oriented, salaried physicians.
4. A surplus of well-educated physicians eager to take less income in order to practice their profession.

5. A marketplace business mentality firmly in place.
6. Fiercely competing companies vying for market shares.
7. The effective loss of the force of the idea of health care as a right, of equal access for all to health care, despite the incredible gains toward the policy objective of health for all during the past twenty-five years.
8. The successful dismantling of much of the central planning and regulatory apparatus, perhaps forever.
9. The progressive growth in numbers of people with no or inadequate health insurance coverage and the swelling ranks of the poor, producing an increase in hospital failures.
10. The growing specter of serious rationing in order to prevent the continual erosion of the gross national product by expenditures for health care.

6

TRAGIC CHOICES
AND THE
POSTMODERN
PARADIGM

"On Nantucket we never mention the Essex."

In his analysis of modern British politics, Professor Sam Beer of Harvard identifies as his real object of concern the sentiments and images that serve as a society's or an institution's or a community's operative ideals. While recognizing that there is no one-to-one correlation between theory and practice, he strongly avers the importance of the political culture of values, beliefs, and emotional symbols in the determination of behavior. "Politics," says Beer, "is a struggle for power, but a struggle that is deeply conditioned by fundamental moral concerns" (1982: xiv).

In dealing with the modernization of British politics, Professor Beer, admittedly drawing heavily upon Max Weber, identifies rationalization and voluntarism as the critical concepts. He defines rationalism as the cultural foundation of the process which allows for the growth of scientific knowledge and the incorporation of its fruits into the society; rationalism is equated then with the values and beliefs defining and supporting the pursuit of scientific knowledge and its use to control the natural and social environment.

Voluntarism is the view that the desires of the people are the basis of legitimacy in constitutional structure and in public policy, in sharp contrast to, for example, the medieval notion that divine command provides the moral authority for civil government. Beer goes on to assert that the enormous proliferation of scientific knowledge characteristic of our postindustrial societies has placed an incredible premium on technical and professional skill. He worries further that the enormous power of mass communication and large-scale survey techniques could place the whole society and its various subsets in the hands of the technocrats who control those venues perhaps to the people's detriment.

Says Professor Beer, "If we are faithful to human appetite as our standard of valuation, we are pretty sure to come out with an equalitarian view of the ultimate foundations of power" (1982: 395). He foresees an increasing concentration of power at the center in the hands of a managerial elite, running large-scale, formal megacorporations, but he worries that all of this could lead to what he calls "pluralistic strangulation," an incapacity to get anything done, a kind of managerial and bureaucratic gridlock. I dwell here at length on Beer's recent analysis of modern British politics because so much of his analysis is pertinent to the health enterprise in America today.

I wish to discuss in this chapter the problem of allocation of scarce resources, but I must first deal in some detail with what the public wants and what I understand about cost control in American health care. In the course of this discussion and that which follows on possible futures for health care, the insights and warnings inherent in Professor Beer's analysis will be apparent.

What then are the American public's appetites, values, and beliefs with regard to health? Any reasonably complete summary is certain to list contradictory ideas and desires for a public so diverse as America's. Individual liberty and freedom of choice along with equal access to essential elements of health care would be prominent on any list. Hope for the individual and the chance for cure or rehabilitation would be at least as important as disease prevention and the promotion of a healthful life-style. There is a strong instinct for people to have their own personal doctors; there is a feeling of dependence upon experts, counselors, and professionals of all sorts to guide one through life's hard spots, such that citizen competence has given way to professional dominance. The American public has been referred to as a pill-taking society and there is certainly a deeply ingrained belief that technology and science can solve most things; there is a tendency to require intervention, to do things to solve problems, to expect new developments and new technological miracles. The last decade has been so productive that no one can blame the public for getting caught up in the technological imperative.

Social critics in the last decade have begun to refer to our society as narcissistic. The health establishment has contributed to this focusing on the individual self by educating the public explicitly or indirectly to believe that health is the highest objective in life. As one wag recently said, it seems as though in America they believe that death is optional; certainly many people expect at least to live pain free and disease free. They believe there should be a way to live free of stress and anxiety. We are taught to be thin and athletic. We expect to live sexually satisfying lives, to have perfect teeth, to feel good about ourselves, and to have a significant proportion of the good things of life. If we are denied any of these things it is deemed tragic. Thus we expect access to all the best in health care and if we don't get it we might sue, and we are suing more often and at greater cost now than ever before, transforming the potentially therapeutic relationship between doctor and patient into an adversarial encounter. The "malpractice crisis," as it is called, is a serious economic problem, but it is much more dangerously destructive to the Hippocratic theme.

On the other side of this coin, there is the rather astonishing growth of self-help, self-care, and health-promoting activities, which all share in a tendency away from the dependence on experts and demonstrate a return to an emphasis on the competent citizen; narcissistic maybe, but at least a competent narcissist!

Finally, the American public has running through it a growing strain of doctor distrust and a belief that it is being charged too much. Thus, as we noted previously, the average patient will change doctors or health care providers if he or she can save $15 per month—so much for the personal physician concept!

Although one may often hear the cliché "The doctor knows best" there is a healthy skepticism about authority and high status and a growing feeling that doctors should be put in their places. Second opinions and competition among specialty groups, despite their duplications and extra expense, fit right into the American scene. The government has reversed financial incentives so as to reduce expenses, but it has so far refused to reduce the physician surplus situation and is only now beginning to make decisions on the basis of cost which could affect quality.

Against this background, let us turn to the issue of allocation of scarce health-related resources or rationing of health services. The efforts to control costs of health care in the United States have progressed in fits and starts. Nowhere has creeping incrementalism been more in evidence than in this sphere. Twenty-five years ago, the problem with rising hospital costs was supposed to be poor management; no one could understand why a hospital room cost so much more than the best hotel and seemed so much worse. That issue got attacked and understood, if not solved. Then it appeared that, in the sixties, the real growth in costs of health care came in the proliferation of thousands of "little ticket" items, such as new laboratory tests and radiologic exams. In the seventies and eighties, the dramatic increases in costs are said to be due mostly to the introduction and diffusion of "big ticket" items like lasers, CAT scans, nuclear magnetic resonance devices, transplants, and other computer-driven advances.

At the same time as our payment systems were encouraging new technologies, experts attempted to estimate the waste resulting from providing unproven tests and treatments. Marcia Angell has recently concluded that the nation's health bill could be cut by 25 percent if we refused to order tests or services of as yet unproven efficacy.

As the bureaucratization developed and the centralization of power, influence, and authority continued to devolve toward the federal government, the latter's approach to cost control ran the gamut from mandatory and voluntary price freezes to planning and regulatory laws requiring, for example, prior approval for the purchase and installation of any device costing in excess of $100,000. Despite these efforts, the cost of health care continued to rise. The Reagan government has turned this approach around (if not by 180 degrees, then by 135 degrees!) by treating the health care industry just as it would any other business and, in essence, letting the marketplace have its way with the cost, efficiency, effectiveness, and distribution of the product.

Whether or not serious "rationing" of health care is needed now in the United States, whether or not health care should get only 6 percent or 12 percent or 18 percent of the gross national product, there is no doubt that demand far outstrips what we wish to spend on health; therefore choices, often based upon governmental or institutional policies, must be made. Such choices in a democratic society, where adherence to values cannot be required from the top down, must inevitably include tragic choices in the lexicon of Calabresi and Bobbitt and will entail a constant shifting of choices to emphasize values apparently neglected by previous policies. We make these choices now but seldom face them directly, cannot in fact bear to face them as a society. How many older Americans die alone and with poor care because of inadequate nursing home facilities, a problem which might be completely solved if we reduced our military budget by a finite amount? How many malnourished and underimmunized children in the United States could be made whole if we stopped major, high technology interventionist therapy in patients over seventy-five or even sixty-five years of age? How shall we care for the poor? How shall we control technology? How encourage it? How many specialists will be allowed? How many primary care doctors should there be? How do we organize for equity of access? Who decides when the life-sustaining machine may be turned off or never turned on? Who rations? How much shall we invest in the future, in the basic sciences? How much in the short-term future, in applied research? How much shall we invest in children, that they may all have a fair chance to compete? How much in "hope," that a trauma center with rehabilitation backup might be available to all who might need it? How much of our GNP should go toward health care? Of that, how much for sick care? How much for prevention? How do we design a system of care allowing for time flexibility so that physicians can be charitable with themselves toward their patients? How do we protect the essentials of the therapeutic relationship—the physician's role as chief patient advocate—without fear of losing pay or job? How shall we pay the doctor? What incentives? (The best element of fee-for-service is that only the patient pays the doctor, so the patient is in control.)

In order to exemplify some of the problems we shall be facing as we attempt to answer these questions over the next five years, I would like to present six brief vignettes or snapshot illustrations. The first occurred in 1960, when as a first-year medical student I had the privilege of watching the great Dr. Robert Gross perform one of his pioneering operations to correct a heart defect in a tiny infant otherwise consigned to an early death. The operation was made possible by the development of the external heart-lung bypass device, the so-called pump-oxygenator, which allowed for pumping and oxygenating the blood for the time required by the surgeon to repair the heart's congenital defect. When Dr. Gross was finished with the repair, the baby's heart and lungs were hooked up again and instantaneously a baby that had been a weird deep blue color became miraculously pink. It was difficult not to break out in applause or tears of joy at that moment. With us in the observation room was a handful of visiting Russian doctors; when Dr. Gross's colleague entered our chamber to greet the visitors they congratulated him but told him that in Russia they would just have a new baby! I remember my deep revulsion at that comment and at a social order that could promote it and felt keenly how important were hope for the downtrodden, a second and possibly a third and fourth chance, and the preciousness of an individual life to us. Now, however, I often wonder whether we are not drawing closer to that 1960 Russian's attitude.

The second example is the recent story of a nine-month terminal hospitalization which produced a bill of $750,000 and incredible hardships for all concerned, most particularly, certainly, the patient. In brief, it began with a hospitalization for arterial bypass surgery in one leg. Complications developed: first there came a series of amputations of the leg, each a little higher as the bypass failed; the patient required surgery for an abdominal obstruction, a tracheotomy and intubation to insure adequate respiration, and, at one point, a several-day drug-induced coma to allow painful debridement of extensive wounds. All of this against a background of a large family which included a doctor and a nurse, with the surgeons, hospital nursing staff, and other well-meaning physician specialists all inserting themselves in the decision-making or decision-influencing loop, frequently with conflicting advice. In the end, the patient was in the hospital, most often in the intensive care unit, at the age of seventy, for the last nine months of her life in a situation no one believed was best. She was kept in her predicament because the hospitalization offered hope for getting her home for some period of comfortable life. One or another of the forces enumerated above acted to prevent the consensus necessary to terminate extraordinary interventions, thus prolonging her treatment. (It should be noted here that approximately 40 percent of all Medicare costs are generated during the last year of life.)

This illustration raises the issue of the quality of the life that has been saved. For many years, critical thinkers about health care have been unhappy with the fact that mortality figures are all too often the only tool available for measuring our health status and the effectiveness of our treatments and interventions. Experts have long sought some measure of the quality of the life preserved; recently such a measure has begun to take shape. It has a catchy new name, is being discussed on both sides of the Atlantic, and, although it remains years away from full applicability, it is already entering into serious thinking about rationing. Our new unit of measure is called the Quality Adjusted Life Year (QALY) and it deserves a brief description here. A single QALY represents a year of life of good quality. Thus, if the average hip replacement allows the recipient ten years of independent mobility, the operation is accorded ten QALY units. One can then divide the cost of the operation by the number of QALY units it produces to get a cost of hip replacement per QALY unit obtained. As this analysis is extended to more and more interventions, so can comparisons be extended of the relative cost of these interventions. Thus, according to the recent work of Professor Maynard of York University, the funds necessary to provide 1 QALY for a chronic renal failure patient will purchase 26 QALYs for patients with immobilizing hip disease and 119 QALYs for smokers cured of their addiction by the educational efforts of their physician. One can immediately see how interesting and useful this sort of information can and will be; it focuses one, for example, upon the cost effectiveness of certain prevention efforts in reducing the burden of illness on a society compared with the cost of therapeutic, high-technology interventions. On the other hand, such figures invite the all-too-easy conclusion that we must always opt for those choices which provide the population with the most QALYs for the money. This, I submit, is a conclusion that should not be accepted without the most serious and probing ethical analysis.

The third example has to do with kidneys and hearts (and I suppose livers and pancreases) and public policy. It was the landmark Social Security legislation of 1965 which broke the stranglehold of the American Medical Association on health policy and established Congress (or the public) as the leader. It did so by extending health insurance to people over sixty-five years of age (Medicare) and to the poor and destitute (Medicaid). In 1972, near the end of the legislative season, Wilbur Mills, then powerful head of the House Ways and Means Committee, allowed a chronic renal failure patient to receive a dialysis treatment at the committee meeting during a hearing on the Medicare budget. The committee learned how these patients could be restored to productive life at a reasonable price (which turned out to be underestimated manyfold) and they voted to do violence to the entire concept of Social Security by extending its largess for the first time to cover treatment for people of all ages with renal failure. They gave, in essence, a blank check to a variety of approaches to the treatment of chronic renal failure. For-profit corporations developed, individuals and groups of doctors made fortunes, and the technology was diffused at great cost very effectively across the population.

Now we have heart transplants entering the realm of clinical effectiveness, but there has been much feeling against approving this procedure for reimbursement by Medicare or any third-party payer. It seems such a drastic procedure; so many, many people would be candidates; the costs would be, one would think, prohibitive if we allowed universal and equal access to this technology. Thus there has been a period of foot dragging about this. This year, it appears the government will pay for heart transplants done at ten centers in the United States.

Economist Roger Evans recently (1986) dealt with this subject, pointing out that, in the first place, a heart transplant and its associated care is not as expensive as some other already approved interventions. Evans prices a heart transplant at from

$80,000 to $110,000 for the first year and $23,000 per year thereafter. These figures compare with the following:

total parenteral nutrition	$110,000 per year
maintenance hemodialysis	$25,000 per year
major adolescent psychiatric disease	$185,000 per case
AIDS treatment	$40,000 to $140,000 per case
bone marrow transplant	$100,000 per case
60 percent burn	$100,000 per case
CABG (coronary artery bypass surgery)	$25,000 per case

Secondly, Evans argues that if it is decided not to reimburse heart transplants, fairness requires that we reexamine all existing reimbursable technical interventions like kidney transplants, bone marrow transplants, and so forth. He argues against holding back on a new technology just because it's newest, saying that kidney patients, for example, should share in the rationing with heart patients rather than denying everything to heart patients just because their replacement therapy was slower in developing.

This third example brings up the entire issue of technology assessment, of the process of bringing the "big ticket" items onto the assembly line, so to speak. Aaron and Schwartz conclude that this is a critical point for cost control once the short-term, one-time benefits of squeezing the fat out of hospital care are realized. How the Western nations, indeed all nations of the world, do this must be the object of intensive study, observation, and comparison in the years ahead. If we bring on expensive new technologies, at least we should purchase those that will be effective, and we must do a far better job of informing the profession and the public about the effectiveness and costs of each one.

The fourth example is a true account of an episode which occurred on February 1, 1821, shortly after the Nantucket whaler *Essex* was sunk in mid-Pacific by an angry bull sperm whale, later forming the basis for Herman Melville's classic, *Moby Dick*. The surviving crew was equally divided among three small boats which set out together for Easter Island; they endured excruciating hardships and eventually were separated from each other in a storm. In one boat, of interest to us here, were Captain Pollard, Barzillai Ray, Charles Ramsdell, young Owen Coffin, who was Captain Pollard's sixteen-year-old nephew, and Samuel Reed, one of the black whalemen.

Captain Pollard's boat and one of the others were still together when the meager supply of food ran out for both boats. And now I quote from Edward A. Stackpole's account in his little book *The Loss of the Essex*.

> At this point, Charles Shorter (an occupant of the second boat), died. For a time they looked at his body. Then, by common consent, they agreed to roast the body and divide it—food.
>
> When Lawson Thomas (also in the second boat) died, the same procedure followed. The resort to human flesh and sinew for food was now the accepted policy among them. When another of the (second boat's) crew, Isaiah Shepard, died, his body was similarly used. A few days later Samuel Reed died in Captain Pollard's boat and the two boat crews shared the body.

On the 28th of January, 1821, a heavy storm drove the two boats apart and (the second) boat was never seen again.

On February 1st, 1821, there was not a scrap of food left in Captain Pollard's boat. A short discussion brought up the alternative that all had avoided up to this moment. But it was voiced at last—one of the five should die—should be killed—to provide food so that his companions might sustain their lives a few more days. The dreaded choice was made by drawing straws. Young Owen Coffin made the fateful draw. Another selection followed—that of the executioner— and Charles Ramsdell found himself cast in that role.

Captain Pollard stood up and looked at his nephew, and recalled saying:

"'My lad! My lad! If you don't like your lot, I will shoot the first man who touches you.' The poor emaciated boy hesitated . . . then quietly laying his head down on the gunnel, he said: 'I like it as well as any other.' He was soon dispatched and nothing of him left. . . . But I can tell you no more. My head is on fire at the recollection: I hardly know what I say!"

Quickly following Captain Pollard's effort to change the fatal decision, Ramsdell, who had become, through the drawing, the executioner, pleaded with Coffin to reverse the procedure—that he might be the victim. But Owen Coffin refused; he had taken the same chance as his shipmates; he had resolved to accept the verdict of the drawing.

The resulting sacrifice must have been a scene the survivors wished to blot from their minds the rest of their lives— were it possible.

What went on among the crew in that tortured little boat during its ninety days at sea must have been in fact an excruciatingly intense examination of great immediacy to the participants of the various issues confronting and options open to those who must deal with the allocation of scarce resources in any setting. If we follow their lead, we shall do something like assign by lot everyone in our population into a graded priority classification, which would then be utilized to determine who would receive, and in what order, limited treatments such as dialysis or organ transplants. The Seattle approach to chronic dialysis was through an anonymous committee deciding on the basis of social utility. Calabresi might say that society couldn't stand the trauma of the constant reminder that it was electing to let people die by random selection, a trauma that the small society of that little boat did elect to tolerate perhaps because they all were so close to death that it might have been appealing to draw the short straw. If perfect justice is to make the allocation decisions on a random basis, then I believe we shall not do so until and unless the constraint in our resource pool becomes so marked that we get a lot closer to the circumstances in that little boat than we are now. Perhaps the strongest evidence in support of my view on this point is reflected in the attitude of Nantucketers themselves regarding the *Essex* and its incredible story. Quoting once more from Stackpole's book: "But on Nantucket neither the principals nor their families could be drawn into a discussion of details. On one occasion, when a historically minded young woman attempted to learn more by questioning a daughter of Benjamin Lawrence, she was kindly but firmly rebuffed. 'Miss Mollie,' she said quietly to her questioner, 'on Nantucket we never mention the *Essex*.'"

The fifth illustration is based upon a study of Princeton theology students published by Darley and Baston in an article entitled "From Jericho to Jerusalem" (1973) wherein senior divinity students were studied for those elements that influenced or produced charitable behavior. Psychological testing was detailed; the critical experiment occurred on a winter day late in the year. The students had to prepare a talk on the parable of the Good Samaritan or on some other subject and were scheduled for individual oral presentations. At the end of a preliminary meeting with a faculty member, the professor informed the student that he or she was already late for the presentation of the talk in a neighboring building (high hurry), or would be right on time if he or she hurried promptly (intermediate hurry), or still had a few minutes to spare but had best be getting over there (low hurry).

In each case, the student encountered a man moaning and groaning with obvious physical distress lying on the grass next to the path, a perfect opportunity to become the modern-day good Samaritan; but many passed him by. On analysis, the one variable among the many tested which correlated positively with those individuals who stopped to give succor was the time available before the next appointment. Personality factors and whether or not the individual had just prepared a talk on the parable of the Good Samaritan did not matter in the decision to stop and help—the availability of time did!

Allow me to juxtapose that study with the plight of a recently graduated obstetrician (our sixth illustration). This lady, a single parent with two relatively young children, was precluded from entering private practice in the city where she lived because she was already $100,000 dollars in debt and couldn't afford the $60,000 required for malpractice insurance. Therefore, she joined a group practice providing prepaid care to a large population of subscribers and was promptly informed by the nonphysician clinic manager that her "quota" was to see five patients per hour. She felt it was impossible to give good care, to adequately educate either pre- or postpartum patients under these circumstances, but she had no alternatives other than quitting. To quit was economic suicide for her and her children and yet she was prevented from rendering to her patients what she regarded as reasonable care. She turned to a senior colleague (and friend of mine) for moral counseling; I wonder what he told her, for this

represents one of the quintessential conflicts of the decade before us as the Hippocratic theme meets the bureaucratic theme
on the playing field of "rationing."

In this situation, the limited resource being allocated is not a
technology but the time necessary to establish and develop a
viable relationship between doctor and patient, and the rationer
is the manager, the person least likely to make the best decision. In the case of doctor time, the doctor, not the manager,
ought to make the rationing decision. Where will it all lead? To
the unionization of doctors, to protect not only their economic
interests but their role as advocates for their patients and the
final arbiters of their own time management as it relates to contact with individual patients?

It is important to clarify what is meant when we say "rationing," because the point can be made that doctors have been rationing all along; some observers don't understand the fuss. For
example, I will agree readily that a doctor in charge of a four-
bed intensive care unit is rationing when he or she chooses the
four sickest patients out of a larger pool of candidates for the
unit. This kind of rationing goes on all the time and is perfectly
consistent from my perspective with the terms implicit in the
doctor-patient relationship. If the doctor chooses the four patients to enter the intensive care unit on grounds other than degree of illness, such as age, employment status, number of de-
pendents, then, in my view, rationing on social rather than
medical grounds is occurring and the doctor should not be the
agent, because such is a betrayal of the patient's trust. Similarly, if a rationing decision is made to turn away a medically
needy patient from the unit despite the availability of empty
beds, the doctor should not be the person to make that decision.
Thus you can see that, from my perspective of the maintenance
of the integrity of the physician-patient relationship, there is rationing that is acceptable for the doctor to do and there is ration-

ing wherein it is unacceptable to have the physician making the actual allocation decision.

In the United Kingdom, the political process makes the macro-decision as to how much money is to be spent but has maneuvered the doctors into the position of rationer (a position which it seems to me may ultimately have devastating effects on the trust between patient and doctor so essential to a healthy transaction). In the United States, the political process has been unable (and I believe will always be unable) to make the rationing decisions necessary to keep the lid on costs; politicians and bureaucrats frequently berate the doctors for not carrying out this function of deciding not to give treatment, despite its availability, to some patients. However, the malpractice courts await those U.S. physicians who deviate from the normal standard. Thus, there is little chance that doctors will be placed in the system as the rationers; nor, in my opinion, should they be so placed, with the exception of that situation surrounding the attempt to have a dignified death. In that situation the doctor may withhold an available therapy not because it is to be saved for someone else, but because such restraint is actually the best treatment for the patient.

Daniel Callahan, the distinguished medical ethicist and director of the Hastings Center, recently (1987) made a brave attempt to address the issue of using age as a criterion for rationing medical technology in the United States. Callahan draws a distinction between "medical age" and "biographical age." He argues that society has no choice but to consider age as a criterion for terminating treatment because of the escalating costs of health care, the inexorable growth of new technologies, and the true requirements of the elderly. Callahan delineates the extraordinary pulls and conflicts upon patients, families, and providers, showing how all are hoisted with the great American petard of fighting to the bitter end and occasionally pulling out a therapeutic victory against all odds. Although many people will agree with Callahan in a general way, he does not produce any compelling logic or argument to drive the reader to accept his conclusion that beyond the late seventies to early eighties treatment goals should be to relieve suffering and promote well-being rather than to stave off death. He proclaims three principles for the medical treatment of the aging: (1) "after a person has lived out a natural life span, medical care should no longer be oriented to resisting death"; (2) "provision of medical care for those who have lived out a natural life span will be limited to the relief of suffering"; (3) "the existence of medical technologies capable of extending the lives of the elderly who have lived out a natural life span creates no presumption whatever that the technologies must be used for that purpose." The later principle of course is reminiscent of that of the pope, who declared in the 1950s that it was not morally required to use extraordinary means to keep a person alive who would die without them. Thus, the pope's statement provided support for the withdrawal of extraordinary life support systems when there was no reasonable hope for life otherwise. Callahan correctly points out that the most difficult, perplexing, even ghastly problem is not why physicians use technology so much, but "why it is so hard to stop using it, even when patient welfare and plain common sense appear to demand just that." He doesn't provide an answer to this most difficult issue, however, and furthermore he gives no indication who is going to be the instrument of his three principles of rationing. Will the rationer be the doctor, the insurance company, the society at large? The issue of stopping a technology once begun is going to require concerted community effort to provide the context in which this behavior will be supported by all concerned. Getting laws in place and rules changed can help, but it is emotion and fear which frequently govern behavior. Getting our health establishment comfortable with discontinuing treatment will be a great achievement.

And now it is time for me to admit defeat, to admit that I too have contracted the Alexis de Tocqueville syndrome (at least a modified form of it), and to pass along my current analysis of what has been for me one of the more perplexing differences between the American and the British practices of medicine. More than a common language separates us. The issue to which I refer was identified in 1963 by the American Nobelist in economics, Kenneth Arrow, when he noted the intrinsic conflict between the doctor as the supplier of services and the doctor as advocate for the patient. Intellectually I understood that statement, but in practice I thought it presented no real problem; therefore, I took it as a rather arcane insight, although somehow I have continued to remember it from time to time. More recently, the American authors Aaron and Schwartz, in their book *The Painful Prescription,* make no bones about their observation that British physicians, both general practitioners and specialists, are making the rationing decisions in certain key instances. The most striking example for an American reader is that of turning down patients for dialysis because of age. I know Bill Schwartz and he is a thoughtful and careful person; I also know several British physicians quite well and they all claimed that they did not make rationing decisions, they made medical decisions. One with many years of practice in London to her credit said she had never had a patient turned down by a specialist. I found it hard to bring these two perceptions of the same phenomena into some sensible alignment until I read of the significant differences between the two countries in the doctrine of informed consent, which was briefly discussed earlier. The informed consent decisions of the American judiciary essentially make the patient the decision maker, not the doctor. It is expected that the doctor presents all the reasonable options to the patient and family; that the authority has become so decentralized that it in effect rests within each patient; that the trust of the patient in the doctor rests upon the latter's demonstrated competence and the honesty and integrity with which he or she deals with the patient.

In the United Kingdom in 1985, the House of Lords, by split vote to be sure, decided the Sidaway case by explicitly denying the informed consent doctrine extant in America and declaring that the patient had a right to hear only what was customary and necessary from the doctor's point of view. Further conversations convince me that most British doctors and patients agree with the implications of the decision. When it is common sense to the doctor that an expensive, extraordinary intervention is unnecessary, it is consistent with the gatekeeper policy for the doctor to simply make that decision for the patient by not recommending referral. In fact, these decisions to the British doctors are medical decisions, whereas to American doctors the very same decision is a rationing decision and not a medical decision. For example, even if American doctors were personally unenthusiastic about putting an elderly patient on chronic dialysis, they would undoubtedly feel that the option must be presented to the patient and that, if the patient chose dialysis, the doctor would be obliged to carry it out. The British patient would be confused by the American physician and the American patient would feel badly shortchanged by the information and choices offered by a British doctor.

It is these thoughts which undergird the view (referred to in Chapter 4) of American economist Charles Begley when he advances from Kenneth Arrow's view of the conflict between physicians as suppliers and advocates to adopt the position that the role of gatekeeper (as in the NHS and in American HMOs) is fundamentally incompatible with the American doctrine of informed consent. I believe the lawyers and the doctors and the policy makers have a lot of hard thinking and negotiating to do on these matters. It is gratifying for me to finally understand how the British doctors and patients have maintained the integrity of their relationship in the face of these tough decisions, but I fear the turbulence which may emerge if the American view of informed consent is adopted in England. Anne Sommers recently pointed out that doctors are now being charged with malpractice for not yielding to patients' wishes to be allowed to die; this suggests that in America the patient may become the rationer! In the end, isn't this where ideas like individual freedom and citizen competence take us?

Thus, the American politicians have turned to the marketplace to do their job for them—and who's to say whether this approach might not have great benefits. This decentralization has had some interesting if unexpected fallout. For example, I have a friend with a complex neurological disorder who is a subscriber to a prepaid comprehensive care plan; when it became clear that he would benefit by having an expensive, new, high-tech intervention to speed his convalescence, he was interviewed by a special group of people not including his doctor to determine whether the plan would purchase it for him or not! This of course is similar to the much-maligned process used in Seattle, Washington, to determine which few patients would get into the chronic dialysis program; the doctors advocated their patients and a board of anonymous lay members made the decisions. The intellectual world scoffed, saying logic and justice required either random selection or universal availability.

Under the deregulated, decentralized systems approach to health care evolving in the United States, the main problem will be how to guarantee a requisite level of care for the poor and underinsured. How we answer that problem will be the true measure of our values, of our national character, and of the quality of our beliefs. If we deal successfully with the issue of the poor and underserved, we may well have achieved an approach to providing adequate health care for all in a context fully supportive of the American values of voluntarism and freedom of choice that may be, for us, better than the more centralized approach we were following toward a single, NHS-like establishment.

A period of confusion, rapid change, and great debate over value-laden issues (such as is now being experienced in the United States regarding health care) cries out for the emergence of philosophers who can clarify issues, define central questions, and help the society toward a rational resolution of the policy crises with which it is dealing. Bona fide card-carrying philosophers have entered this fray and one of them has, in my view, recently published a comprehensive and illuminating analysis which has the potential to help shape and clarify our nation's thinking on some of the crucial health-related questions. I refer to Norman Daniels's treatise published in 1986 by Cambridge University Press, *Just Health Care.* Professor Daniels attempts to extend John Rawls's (1971) principle of distributive justice to health care and courageously attacks the most pressing and difficult issues.

In brief, he argues that health care is of a different order from other commodities or services and that the principle governing health policy should be what he calls "the fair equality of opportunity account," implying that society has the obligation, based upon the Rawlsian theory of justice as fairness, to see to it that each person has access to the health care required to allow him or her equal opportunity as a citizen within the constraints of his or her own innate talents and skills. Daniels further concludes that the arrangements necessary to provide this care would not violate any basic provider liberties and should not necessarily do economic injustice to doctors. In his view, the restrictions on autonomy in treatment decisions derived from just resource allocation policies will not harm the rights of either patients or doctors or the essence of the doctor-patient relationship as long as the society understands its obligation to exclude the rationing decisions from the physician's portfolio of responsibilities.

Although I lay no claim to being a professional philosopher, I commend Professor Daniels's work to you and find in it the best set of arguments I have yet come across yielding some principles for policy development. One hopes his views can gain enough exposure to influence the body politic in a timely fashion.

In a much acclaimed analysis of health care in the United States, Professor Paul Starr, in his book *The Social Transformation of American Medicine,* offers little hope for a true partnership in addressing the problems of the future among the public, the health corporations, and the profession of medicine, a profession led by an army of physicians whom he sees as power and money hungry. Professor Starr's work has been generally praised and has become a runaway best-seller in its field.

In commenting on Professor Starr's book, sociologist Florence A. Rudermann (1986) chided him for demonstrating a methodologic failing she finds common to most medical sociologists; that is, an over-emphasis on external forces when examining medicine and an under-appreciation for science, technology, and the intrinsic values and moral forces of medicine. For her, Starr fails because he describes everything that has gone on in American health care as (1) a natural response by the medical profession to forces external to it and (2) caused by physicians' drive to power and wealth. Rudermann believes that science and technology, two separable entities and forces, create their own values and ideas which often move things, as far as society is concerned, in uncomfortable ways and have had major impacts on health care. Further, she believes the profession of medicine has a powerful tradition and an important and compelling ethos and set of values which have played and continue to play important roles in the shaping of health care. Lastly, she roundly criticizes Professor Starr for his failure to describe the crucial expression through the medical profession and the health care establishment of society's wishes, values, policies, and confessions. Although I believe Starr's book has in fact provided a more balanced perspective than Rudermann attributes to it, I think her points of emphasis on the societal power of the ideas behind science and technology merit our attention.

There are other voices, however, being raised to proclaim the need for a new commitment beyond personal advancement and pleasure. The emptiness and cultural boredom attendant upon our enormous materialistic successes have led more of us on a renewed quest for individual and collective meaning. In a widely acclaimed book, *Habits of the Heart—Individualism and Commitment in American Society*, Robert Bellah and his associates have put their fingers upon the key element for any new paradigm for our society in the postmodern era; that element involves both a sense of community and collective response. As Bellah points out, Alexis de Tocqueville in the middle third of the nineteenth century identified the potential downside for our society of the entrepreneurial utilitarianism of Benjamin Franklin. With the heavy Republican and biblical influences of the early American democracy (as personified by John Winthrop and Thomas Jefferson), a sense of transcendant direction and of societal community was characteristic; but the rugged and utilitarian individualism of Franklin soon engendered some warning signs in Tocqueville's picture of the new republic. The latter described the rise of increasing numbers of people in the young republic whose sense of self-sufficiency so isolated them from the rest of the society that they invariably seemed not to appreciate that they were dependent on others for their existence and success in society. As Bellah quotes Tocqueville, "Individualism is a word recently coined to express a new idea. Our fathers knew only about egoism." Though individualism is more moderate and orderly than egoism, the results on the society are the same, according to Tocqueville.

Individualism is a calm and considered feeling which disposes each citizen to isolate himself from the mass of his fellows and withdraw into the circle of family and friends; with this little society formed to his taste, he gladly leaves the greater society to look after itself. . . . there are more and more people who, though neither rich nor powerful enough to have much hold over others, have gained or kept enough wealth and enough understanding to look after their own needs. Such folk owe no man anything and hardly expect anything from anybody. They form the habit of thinking of themselves in isolation and imagine that their whole destiny is in their hands. Eventually they reach the stage where they also "forget their ancestors" as well as their descendants. "Each man is forever thrown back on himself alone and there is danger that he may be shut up in the solitude of his own heart."

One of the main conclusions of this interpretive study of American life is that what people desperately miss is that sense of community purpose sufficient to draw them together in a self-transcendant common bond. This need must be fulfilled if a constructive and creative postmodern America is to emerge. This same need is felt at all levels of our society and in our institutions. Thus, it would follow that without a greater sense of community and mutual belonging and interconnection, it is unlikely that an optimal plan will emerge for the allocation of scarce health resources or an approach to health services which is reasonably fair and just for all our citizens. Modifying our beliefs and behavior so that personal success and advancement are not our major and overriding goals requires a change in what Tocqueville called our "habits of the heart." If it comes into being, and it will take some time to do so, our habits of the heart will have altered such that we might easily refer to the change as a paradigm shift; if such changes sifted down to health care, we might be able to describe a postmodern paradigm for our health care sector, a paradigm that preserves liberty, freedom, hope, and a sense of human progress which incorporates suffering and death, all united through a sense of belonging and community. As expressed in health care, the postmodern paradigm would successfully intertwine the Hippocratic and bureaucratic themes because they would be subsumed under it.

Although a new postmodern paradigm for our society or for the health sector is far from a reality, its form is taking shape. Our desire to seek purposes beyond our own personal gain should not be underestimated.

In summary, I conclude that in the United States we have in health care what the people want. What the people want varies from time to time, but the values of voluntarism, access to care, hope for a better life, and a second chance for the individual wherever possible will remain basic to whatever we do in the years ahead. Whatever is not based on those values in health policy will not long endure. The very diversity, confusion, and multiplicity of approaches to getting health services to our people express our national character and our desire not to have things controlled for us by people in a far-away place—and for many Americans in 1988, Washington is almost as remote from them as London was to the colonists in 1776.

Rosemary Stevens, the British-born American historian of medicine, has recently observed that whereas England lives according to fairness, America lives according to rules (I know a thoughtful observer who says America lives by getting around the rules). Clearly, fairness in the sense of the adequate provision of health services to all is the top priority in England, and it has been achieved. It is equally clear that fairness is not the top priority in America, although it has been a major national objective; our current course in health policy, if it continues uncorrected, is producing a system which is less and less fair. As that fact becomes increasingly clear to our voting public, and as that public becomes more and more brought together in an enhanced sense of community, the American sense of fairness as regards the provision of health care to everyone may again be felt as a major thrust in our public policy.

Although more money is spent on health care in America on a per capita basis than in any of the other Western democracies, it must be remembered that only 41 percent of those expenditures are from the public treasury, as compared with 80 to 90 percent in other nations. In other words, the United States spends in public funds on health care approximately the same proportion of the GNP as does the United Kingdom. As complicated and difficult as it will be to accomplish, I believe it is time for a dramatically comprehensive rethinking of how America's health-directed public funds are expended. The first priorities should be the poor of any age and coverage of catastrophic illness for the entire population. It is possible that by rethinking our Medicare program and our other publicly funded entities we might more effectively address our most pressing problems of providing access for everyone to health services of a higher standard. As we seek a competent citizenry through a wide variety of social strategies, perhaps we should especially focus health promotion and disease prevention programs on the poor and socially disadvantaged. The AIDS epidemic will turn the social spotlight more onto public health measures in the decade ahead rather than on technological interventions for cure. The possibilities for reform are endless; admittedly the difficulties and obstacles to such corrective actions seem almost infinite, but the time for America to settle these questions is at hand. The poet's warning will be heeded that the future of the nation is foretold by the manner in which it treats those creatures that cannot do for themselves, but it will in all likelihood not be perfectly heeded and we will be haunted by those inequities. Like the Nantucketers, we shall continue to have our *Essex*es, and we won't like to talk about them. The Bellahs of the nation will continue to remind us that our biblical and Republican forefathers were deeply concerned for the society if there are excessive gaps between the rich and the poor and that Ben Franklin's "God helps those who help themselves" philosophy contains the seeds of despair for a free society.

For the rest of the system, my guess is that creeping incrementalism will hold true—that our system will have been tilted toward competition, that money will be made, but that for-profit chains will not dominate. Further, the continuing surfeit of physicians will lead to a decrease in physicians' incomes and will fuel large group enterprises which will vie for patients; professional-technical competence will remain a critical factor, with price competition built around creature comforts and amenities. Holistic approaches will be incorporated into Western practice—doctors will again touch patients, may even learn to relax their muscles through manipulation (or will have such therapists on their immediate team), and through talking and listening will encourage their patients' trust and confidence in their own capacities to improve with the assistance of a physician-scientist of high competence. More and more medical care will move out of the hospital and into the ambulatory setting, leaving the hospital for intensive care and rehabilitation. Costs will continue to increase, but we shall spend more on prevention, rehabilitation, and chronic disease than is now the case. Technology assessment will be on firmer and more rational grounds as the complexities of cost-benefit analyses at last yield to the intelligence of economists and policy makers. We shall tilt more toward primary care within multispecialty groups, and primary care will emphasize prevention to a greater degree.

The large health care company can become humane, can project competence, concern, and compassion, and those that do will succeed, but we shall preserve the individual's right to choose by providing diversity even at greater cost. I believe, in fact, that though considerably shrunken, the private fee-for-service sector will remain an important part of the enterprise.

For the past thirty years, our nation's medical schools have attracted the very best students; it is obvious that to sustain and further develop the excellence of our health care, we need to sustain that supply of talented young people, even if we jiggle with the number from time to time. One of the troublesome aspects of the current period of uncertain flux is the increasingly negative attitude toward the practice of medicine on the part of the doctors themselves. Although convincing data are hard to come by, many observers believe this to be the case on an empirical basis. For example, a survey of my twenty-fifth reunion medical school class showed that a mere handful of us were of a mind to vigorously encourage our children to go into medicine.

Much of this ambiguity may be attributable to the change in public attitude toward the doctor as director to the doctor as junior partner and to the changes inherent in going from individual solo practices to more complicated and bureaucratic arrangements. I believe that one of the most deleterious and correctable negative forces is the malpractice situation. When premiums in some states for some practitioners rise to six figures, we find doctors dropping out or refusing, for example, to deliver babies. A system that was designed for useful social purposes no longer adequately achieves many of them. People who are wronged get some of the jury awards while the lawyer pockets a major portion; the whole society pays the bill insofar as the costs of malpractice insurance are spread among all the patients or insured population. All too often, patients who should receive some compensation neither ask for nor receive any, because lawsuits aren't their style or because they like their doctor. Alternatively, patients who do file suit may or may not have been treated incompetently, but in most cases the doctor has done a poor job of communicating. The settlements awarded by juries are often ludicrously large and even a few such aberrations raise the rates for everyone for protection against such possibilities. There are alternatives; there is a serious debate going on which seems to me to be going currently in no particular direction.

Meanwhile the doctor-patient relationship is being eroded progressively; the necessary trust can never develop when a latent and not so latent adversarial relationship is behind every encounter. For the sake of argument, if I were given the power to decide the issue right now, I would limit the size of total settlements, limit the percentage of the lawyer's take to no more than 10 percent, and make a serious effort to develop a no-fault compensation plan which would divide a fixed pool of dollars among the injured. The British have no juries for malpractice litigation and there are those who say that such a change might solve most of our problems. There seems little doubt that a national health insurance program would significantly reduce the malpractice, medical liability problem, because patients and family would know that all health care costs would be covered; only "pain and suffering" would remain. Thus, if the matter goes unresolved, it could become a strong force in pushing the country toward a program of national health insurance.

I do not believe that the procompetition movement in health care is intrinsically nefarious, that the rise of the for-profit chains is destructive, that the treatment of health care as an industry or business is necessarily bad. Although perhaps not the most desirable approach from all points of view, I think the so-called industrialization of medicine is as much a challenge as a threat; a fruitful and creative matrix of the for-profit entities with the traditional health care systems, the public and not-for-profit hospitals can emerge to sustain American health care at a very high level for all our people. An important element in such a happy outcome must be a medical profession that remains firmly rooted in its Hippocratic tradition, that refuses to budge from the crucial tenets of its code of ethics, that manages to maintain its independence, that develops and implements the core ideas that have for centuries guided the best efforts of a healing profession based on scientific observation and method.

I believe this means that, just as our biomedical sciences

continue to produce new curative technological interventions, just as our social and behavioral sciences develop new strategies to encourage life-style changes in healthful directions, so the medical profession should extend its intellectual boundaries to include the fuller exploration and understanding of the therapeutic relationship or, if you will, healing. Anthropology and psychology can, in my view, forge a constructive, productive linkage with the neurosciences (including neuropharmacology) to extend our knowledge in this important area. Along the way, we must continue to ask the question, "How can the physician be the patient's friend and trusted advocate while being a potential adversary and rationer at the same time?"

In other words, I believe an accommodation can be reached between the values of the Hippocratic theme and those of the bureaucratic theme, that physicians will be sorely tested to remain true to their core values, but that if they do and if the public provides a mechanism (through taxation and public funds) to finance high quality care for the unemployed and otherwise underserved, then America will at last have expressed its basic values more completely than is now the case through its health care delivery apparatus. Thus, though I applaud the courage, energy, and wit of those who are attacking the bureaucratic windmill as it is expressed in the procompetitive movement, I think they are charging the wrong windmill. Although history may declare the effort equally quixotic, the windmill I have marked for attack is the one that houses forces within and without the medical profession which would destroy the modern expression of the Hippocratic theme, that would, in my view of things, destroy the core of the profession.

To preserve a healing profession with its roots in the science and commitment of the Hippocratic tradition, we must be clear that the patient's and the public's interests are primary; the health professions and the entire health industry will have to prove this commitment to the society which nurtures them. If we can manage to produce a new amalgamation of our basic values into a postmodern paradigm, we may, in fact, have opened the way for the full expression of healing professions and healing people within a healing society—a worthy goal that can keep us all constructively busy for the foreseeable future.

How will it all come out? I don't know, but I believe we all will know by 1995. I anticipate with confidence and hope that calmer, more serene time when scholars in the year 2000 will be able to present the full story with the accuracy afforded by a reasonable historical perspective. Until then, however, since I am certain only of our uncertainties and that I can ask more questions than I can answer, I look forward to continuing transnational dialogue in the years to come as the United Kingdom and the United States, along with other Western democracies, attempt to deal with justice, fairness, and cost control issues in an enterprise centered around high technology and healing. The continuing challenges to the evolution of health policy in the modern, postindustrial Western democracy or voluntary society are great indeed. We shall continue to need cross-cultural analyses of progress almost as much as we need a heightened sense of purpose and community.

REFERENCES

Aaron, Henry J., and William B. Schwartz. *The Painful Prescription* (Washington, D.C.: Brookings Institution, 1984).

Adams, Francis. *The Genuine Works of Hippocrates* (Huntington, N.Y.: Robert E. Krieger, 1972).

Beer, Samuel H. *Modern British Politics—Parties and Pressure Groups in the Collectivist Age* (Great Britain: Faber and Faber, 1982).

Begley, Charles. "Prospective Payment and Medical Ethics." *Journal of Medicine and Philosophy* 12 (1987): 107–122.

Bellah, Robert N., Richard Madsen, William M. Sullivan, Anne Swidler, and Steven M. Tipton. *Habits of the Heart—Individualism and Commitment in American Life* (New York: Harper and Row, 1985).

Bok, Sissela. *Lying and Moral Choice* (New York: Random House, 1979).

Brewster, Kingman. "The Voluntary Society." In *The Tanner Lectures on Human Values*, vol. 4 (Salt Lake City: University of Utah Press, 1983), pp. 1–41.

Calabresi, Guido, and Philip Bobbitt. *Tragic Choices* (New York: W. W. Norton, 1978).

Califano, Joseph A. *America's Health Care Revolution* (New York: Random House, 1986).

Callahan, Daniel. "Terminating Treatment: Age as a Standard." *Hastings Center Report* 17, no. 5 (October–November 1987): 21–25.

Dahrendorf, Ralph. *Life Chances: Approaches to Social and Political Theory* (London: Weidenfeld and Nicholson, 1979).

References

Daniels, Norman. *Just Health Care* (Cambridge: Cambridge University Press, 1986).

Darley, John M., and C. Daniel Baston. "From Jericho to Jerusalem—A Study of Situational and Dispositional Variables in Helping Behavior." *Journal of Personality and Social Psychology* 27 (1973): 100–108.

Derthick, Martha, and Paul Quirk. *The Politics of Deregulation* (Washington, D.C.: Brookings Institution, 1985).

Ducker, Thomas B. "We Need a Cure for the Lack of Medical Trust." *Houston Chronicle*, February 2, 1987, op-ed page.

Erikson, Erik. "The Golden Mean in the Cycle of Life." In R. J. Bulger, ed., *In Search of the Modern Hippocrates* (Iowa City: University of Iowa Press, 1987).

Evans, Roger W. "The Heart Transplant Dilemma." *Issues in Science and Technology* (Spring 1986): 91–101.

Handlin, Oscar. *The Uprooted*, 2d ed. (Boston: Atlantic–Little, Brown, 1973).

The Institute for Medicine. *For-profit Enterprise in Health Care* (Washington, D.C.: National Academy Press, 1986).

Jennett, Bryan. *High Technology Medicine: Benefits and Burdens* (New York: Oxford University Press, 1986).

Katz, Jay. *The Silent World of Patient and Doctor* (New York: Free Press, 1984).

Kleinman, Arthur. *Patients and Healers in the Context of Culture* (Berkeley and Los Angeles: University of California Press, 1980).

Lain Entralgo, Pedro. *The Therapy of the Word in Classical Antiquity* (New Haven: Yale University Press, 1970).

Majno, Guido. "The Lost Secret of Ancient Medicine." In R. J. Bulger, ed., *In Search of the Modern Hippocrates* (Iowa City: University of Iowa Press, 1987).

Merton, Thomas. *Love and Living*, ed. Naomi Burton Stone and Brother Patrick Hart (San Diego and New York: Harcourt Brace Jovanovich, 1979).

Ornstein, Robert, and David Sobel. *The Healing Brain* (New York: Simon and Schuster, 1987).

Rawls, John. *A Theory of Justice* (Cambridge, Mass.: Harvard University Press, 1971).

Reiser, Stanley J., and Michael Anbar. *The Machine at the Bedside* (Cambridge: Cambridge University Press, 1984).

Richards, Dickinson W. "Hippocrates and History: The Arrogance of Humanism." In R. J. Bulger, ed., *In Search of the Modern Hippocrates* (Iowa City: University of Iowa Press, 1987).

Rudermann, Florence A. "A Misdiagnosis of American Medicine." *Commentary* 81, no. 1 (January 1986): 43–49.

Starr, Paul. *The Social Transformation of American Medicine* (New York: Basic Books, 1973).

Tancredi, Laurence R., and Lola Romanucci-Ross. "The Anthropology of Healing." In R. J. Bulger, ed., *In Search of the Modern Hippocrates* (Iowa City: University of Iowa Press, 1987).

White, Hayden. *Metahistory* (Baltimore, Md.: Johns Hopkins University Press, 1974).

White, Theodore. "The American Idea." *New York Times Magazine*, July 6, 1986, p. 13.